For [illegible], [illegible]

winter,

Greg

NB p210 has been
transposed.

Diary of a
Vagabond Therapist

Other Books by the Same Author

(Ed.) *Modern Manual Therapy of the Vertebral Column* (Edinburgh, Churchill Livingstone, 1986).

Common Vertebral Joint Problems, 2nd edn (Edinburgh, Churchill Livingstone, 1988).

Mobilisation of the Spine, 5th edn (Edinburgh, Churchill Livingstone, 1991).

Diary of a Vagabond Therapist

by

Gregory P. Grieve

The Pentland Press Ltd
Edinburgh · Cambridge · Durhàm · USA

First published in 1998 by
The Pentland Press Ltd.
1 Hutton Close
South Church
Bishop Auckland
Durham

British Library Cataloguing in Publication Data.
A catalogue record for this book is available
from the British Library.

ISBN 1 85821 600 1

Typeset by George Wishart & Associates, Whitley Bay.
Printed and bound by Bookcraft Ltd., Bath.

Contents

List of Illustrations

Illustration Credits
(AC = Author's Collection)
1-3 AC, 4 Dent and Sons, 5, 6, 7 AC, 8 F.D. Ommaney, 9
RAF Museum 10, 11, 12, 13, 14, 15 AC, 16, 17, 18, 19, 20,
21, 22, 24 Imperial War Museum, 23 Hutchinson, 25 Hollis
and Carter, 26 AC, 27 Hutchinson, 28, 29 AC, 30, 31, 32
Hollis and Carter, 33, 34, 35, 36 AC.

Permission to reproduce figures, granted by Dent and Sons,
F.D. Ommaney's executors, the RAF Museum, Hendon
and the Imperial War Museum, Lambeth, is gratefully
acknowledged.

Note. Every effort has been made to trace the owners of
copyright and where successful, permission to reproduce has
been sought and obtained. To those who were untraceable
after the lapse of fifty years, I offer my apologies and trust
that they will allow the indulgence of the odd reproduction.

G.P. Grieve

Preface

Now nearing the end of my days, it occurred to me that a short account of my life and times might be of interest to others. This notion was fostered by contemporaries, who have urged me to put the account on paper. Here it is then, a boyhood in Rhodesia (1919-34), fifteen years in the Royal Navy (1934-48), including the war years and the *Bismarck* and other actions at sea, training as a physiotherapist (1949-52) and physiotherapy teacher (1961-3), specializing in manipulative therapy, and the final years of clinical teaching and authorship.

I have been a very lucky man – I had a lovely wife and forty-six years of happily married life.

Other than alterations of names, this is a true account.

Acknowledgements

I am grateful to Hugh Phillips BSc (Hons) MB FRCS, Consultant Orthopaedic Surgeon, in whose agreeable company, both at the Royal National Orthopaedic Hospital in London in times past, and more recently at the Norfolk and Norwich Hospital, I have learned much. He has kindly honoured me by writing the Foreword to this book.

I express my thanks to John Tydeman, Medical Photographer of the Norfolk and Norwich Hospital, for his unvarying technical excellence and devoted skill in getting the best out of somewhat faded old illustrations. Also to Angela Sheffield, for typing the elegant fair copy of my manuscript. I also express my thanks to Arms and Armour Press, for permission to quote from Appendix 3: '*Rodney*'s gunnery action with the *Bismarck*'.

I give thanks, too, for my shipmates of fifty and sixty years ago. They remain in my memories and affections, and I am grateful for the good fellowship we enjoyed. Many of them went down during the War – may their merry souls rest in peace.

CHAPTER I

Early Years

One of a trio of British SE5a aeroplanes, flying above the trenches of Flanders on an early autumn morning in 1918, was piloted by my father, Flight Lieutenant Basil Edward Grieve. Born among the Kimberley diamond diggings of Scottish parents in 1887, he fostered his interest in geology and had become a mining compound manager in the Rhodesian goldfields before coming to England in 1915 to join the Army and 'do his bit', like so many young men from overseas. Subsequently, he transferred from the Machine-gun Corps to the Royal Flying Corps, thereby planting in me the seed of my lifelong passionate love affair with biplanes – 'proper' aeroplanes. So far as I am concerned, the jet engine and the monoplane have sent aviation to the dogs. I mean, without the wind singing in the flying wires and the sun glinting on the doped fabric covering the silver wings, where are you?

After demobilization, my father remained in England, by which time he had gathered a wife and two sons – Geoffrey born on 18 August 1917 and myself born on 11 December 1918. But Africa was in his blood, as any old Africa hand would tell you, and in 1921 he took his new wife and the two little boys back to Salisbury, Southern Rhodesia (now

Harare, in Zimbabwe). Hence my earliest memories are not of England but of the Rhodesian savannah or the Mashonaland 'high veldt', an extensive plateau some 5,000 feet above sea level. I cannot say I was impressed – I just did not like Africa. My dislike of Africa was strengthened by a spell of four years (1929-33) at St George's College (Fig. 1), an imposing edifice devoted to the austere Jesuit education of young Rhodesian boys, plus Catholics from neighbouring Portuguese East Africa (now Mozambique) and South Africa. The excellent teaching, which included French, Latin and Greek from quite early on, was enforced with a certain muscular Roman Catholicism, and underpinned by liberal use of the cane and lots of attendances at chapel and the confessional. More than once I suffered the strong right arm of Father McQuillan as he applied six of the best to my cringing backside. He was known bitterly as 'Tortoise' McQuillan because he applied the strokes so slowly. Father

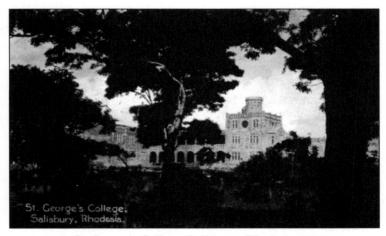

1. St George's College, Salisbury, Rhodesia 1933.

('Machine Gun') Thompson was much more popular as he laid on the six with the rat-a-tat of a Lewis gun.

On 12 April 1922 a third son was born to my parents in Salisbury – Phil had joined the party.

As a young English wife, an Anglican, in a new and alien subtropical environment, my mother longed annually to see again the spring daffodils, to smell the sweet scents of summer and enjoy the misty, mellow fruitfulness of autumn and the Christmas snow. In 1926 she did. Late that year my father obtained leave of absence from Salisbury Town House, where he was then working in the Department of Mines. He sent my mother and the boys ahead of him to her parent's home in West Byfleet, Surrey – and we stayed in Byfleet for five months. But the strong, subtle pull of Africa had entered her blood too, and thereafter, whether in Salisbury or Surrey (which she twice was) she hankered to be in the other place.

We boys were agog with excitement at the prospect of getting on the train for Cape Town and the boat for England – of which I could recall nothing, of course. The slow, five-day railway journey from Salisbury to Cape Town was a thing to be remembered for always, since there was such romance in 'Rhodesian Railways' of those days. For as long as I could remember, the arrival of the boat train from Cape Town had been a social occasion of some importance – like Ascot or the Henley Regatta. Travel was a much more serious and important undertaking than the hyper-convenient 'packaged' travelling of today. We used to go down to the station to see the weekly boat train come in, on Sundays if my memory is sound, if only to look at the new faces of people who had been in England only the month before. There was always the faint and exciting chance of meeting an acquaintance from the UK. The thought of actually boarding that train and making that awesome journey back to England filled the whole of my seven-year-old imagination.

The South African Republic possesses a narrow-gauge railway system with almost the heaviest traffic and the finest rolling stock in the world. This is not a new development, for South Africa and Rhodesia (Zimbabwe) have a tradition of luxury travel. In 1902 Cecil Rhodes introduced the Zambesi Express De Luxe, between Bulawayo and Cape Town; its twelve bogie coaches included a buffet car into which was squeezed a library and reading room, a writing room, a card room, a smoking room and finally an observation balcony – wine coolers, crimson leather and electric light added to the decor. Equally luxurious, and offering the amenity of hot and cold showers, were the Cape Town boat trains. South African long distance 'expresses' may not be fast – the very best do little more than an average of 40 m.p.h. – but this is inseparable from the narrow 3'6" gauge. Some of them rank as truly great trains, running through country which is wild and sometimes splendid and aiming high in matters of comfort. The South African 'Blue Train', for example, covering close on a thousand miles from Johannesburg to Cape Town twice weekly, in some twenty-five hours, was inaugurated a little over four decades ago, when it seemed plain that the future lay only with the aeroplane. The 'Blue Train' was re-equipped in the early seventies with new coaches, carrying no more than about 100 passengers who were served by a staff of twenty-six. Where there are no separate sleeping cars, first- and second-class passengers are given fold-down bunks. It was in such a compartment that my mother shepherded her herd of small boys from Salisbury to Cape Town.

4

I recall little of that seemingly interminable five-day railway ride, other than my huge delight at the novelty of lying in my pyjamas and watching the early morning scenery pass by the compartment window. There were exciting railway bridges, gorges and mountains, and rivers far below, with the occasional unspecified wild animals, herds of this and that, to look at. There were interesting strong points, relics of the long and bloody Boer War, only a quarter of a century before. I recall Bulawayo and its intense heat, De Aar, Kimberley, the Hex river, the Orange river and endless expanses of bush, burning in the sun. Then at Cape Town we saw the sea! I was astonished and terrified by this prodigious expanse of water, with the sun shining on the white horses, the salt wind, the screaming, wheeling gulls and the great looming side of the Union Castle liner, as our train entered the dock area. I knew what ships looked like but had never been so close to one, that I could recall.

I was a very imaginative child, and often saw horrors and delights where there were none. I was nearly wetting myself with excitement and anxiety for our safety at the prospect of that perilous journey to England. Confidence was restored when we had settled ourselves into our cabin, with its main bed for Mother and bunk beds for us boys. We marvelled at the interesting fittings and it began again to become high adventure. The boat was a further delight, especially that lovely romantic smell of ships. We soon became good sailors and rattled our way confidently along the passageways and up and down the stairways.

I still have total recall of a tall, moustachioed man in a brown pinstripe suit and a check tweed cap. He became rather persistent. My mother was then a handsome full-busted woman of thirty-one, and as there was no husband in evidence this Lothario thought he was onto a good thing, no doubt. After my mother had conversed politely with him during a couple of deck meetings, he seemed to have shown his hand. I do not know what Mother said but her rejoinder plainly took the wind out of his sails forthwith. He kept a respectful distance after that and bothered us no more. There was always something exciting to wonder at – flying fishes, porpoises playing around the ship, frequently-seen spouting whales while south of the equator, and the lovely, endless expanse of sea, with the snow-white curling tops of the waves endlessly falling back into the green-blue glittering surface of the water. Even after countless journeys by sea, and some fifteen years in the Navy, that wind-blown ballet of the great waters never fails to fascinate me.

As we sailed past the Canary Islands we were put out at the complete absence of canaries – not one to be seen anywhere. A real let-down. We leant on the guard rails and gazed at Madeira like old seagoing hands, by now itching for the next stop which was Southampton. The meeting at Southampton, the welcome from my maternal grandparents and the prospect of yet another train journey, this time by Southern Railway to West Byfleet, put a cap on the excitement of this high adventure.

To youngsters who had, in effect, known only the high veldt, the comparatively dry, scrubby bush of Rhodesia, England was a fairyland, a knockout of lovely surprises – or so it was to me. I cannot recall my brothers' reaction but I suppose there were much the same as my own, although I do know now that Geoff and Phil both hated the cold and the damp. I found enchanting the wooded greenery of Surrey, the holly trees and the frost and the snow, and the tangy smell of the railway engine smoke. My grandparents, of sturdy Surrey/Hampshire peasant stock, lived near the railway. He was a Southern Railway signalman, and very proud of it, too. In those days, everybody looked up to engine-drivers and signalmen since they held positions of great importance and responsibility; they were highly esteemed by the townspeople. Going down to the woods with my grandfather to collect leaf mould for his potato patch was a delightful adventure, and being invited up to the signal box to watch him pull the great levers was a special treat. I was fascinated, too, by the rather dull-looking birds, by their extraordinary tameness. After the raucous calls of the multi-coloured African birds it was pure enchantment to listen to the sweet blackbirds and thrushes.

School had to continue, of course, and I don't recall any difficulty in blending in among the boys and girls in the playground and classrooms of West Byfleet school. It was certainly co-educational, all right. Behind my desk sat a snub-nosed little Jezabel who seemed set on getting me to admire the holes in her knickers. She would tap me on the shoulder with her ruler, and if I then ducked down and looked behind I'd see she had her little thighs wide open, revealing her torn and grubby underwear. I don't recall any erotic excitement, only astonishment at this forward young miss – but I always did look, of course. Attachments of the heart were directed elsewhere, to none other than Trixie Whitlock, whose apple cheeks and elegant ankles I can visualize to this day. I used to wait by the short walkway tunnel under the railway at the station and carry her satchel home for her. I really do believe she reciprocated my feelings, to a degree anyway. On Boat Race day 1927 she tied a dark-blue ribbon to the handlebars of my little bicycle – I have stoutly supported Oxford ever since. Even in those days, West Byfleet was essentially a dormitory town for many London doctors (particularly from St Thomas's Hospital, near Waterloo station), stockbrokers lawyers and the like, and there were quite a number of motorcars about, as well as the obligatory Sainsbury's, of course. It was considered very grown-up to throw pine cones at the cars and then scuttle behind the nearest hedge.

My passion for biplanes was amply fed, since Weybridge and thus Brooklands aerodrome (and the Vickers aircraft construction shed) were close by. A common and exciting spectacle was the lumbering take-off of twin-engined Vickers Virginia biplane bombers, which used to roar over Byfleet as they slowly gained height. Curiously those antiquated biplanes were in service from 1924 to 1937. Their top speed was only 108 m.p.h. yet they equipped front-line bomber squadrons for several years after the RAF had raised the world speed record to over 400 m.p.h. with the highly streamlined Supermarine SB6 racing monoplane seaplanes.

On turning right after leaving the house, and going down the road called Sherewater, one passed on the left a large thatched house – Oldway. Two or three years ago I went to Byfleet to attend a funeral and took a nostalgic walk around that charming old byway. The wooded area opposite Oldway had been cleared long before to make way for a housing estate, but the old thatched house was still there, as I had remembered it. At the bottom of Sherewater was the bridge over the Basingstoke canal, which meandered along from Byfleet to Woking. It was very much in use in those days, with considerable barge traffic, and it was common to see a large muscular horse plodding along the towpath and pulling a laden barge of coal. The canal was wonderfully quiet and tranquil – after the horses had passed everything settled down again and the moorhens stopped fluttering about. The towpath made a marvellous walk from Byfleet to Woking and back.

Curiously, I cannot recall any special events in that time up to spring and early summer of 1927, except the arrival of my father in December. The family was made whole just in time for Christmas and it was truly beautiful to watch my mother and father embrace; he still wearing greatcoat and hat. Our joy was complete and the angels sang.

Then came the devastating news that we were to return to Salisbury in the late spring. The days and weeks flew by with dreadful speed, until we were once again on the train for Southampton – for me, with a heavy heart. I resolved I'd get back to England as soon as I could but events dictated otherwise and there seemed no prospect of a return. My father's eventful life was cut short at the tragically early age of forty-three, in 1930, the death certificate testifying to acute lobar pneumonia and cardiac failure. There were no antibiotics then and one survived that killer disease by luck only, although good nursing helped. My mother died young, too, but lived long enough to know that her three sons had survived the war at sea, which still pleases me. She was fifty-one when she succumbed in 1946 while under general anaesthesia for a hysterectomy. She too, would have survived today, of course. She was laid to rest in the hot, alien soil of Salisbury cemetery, not far from the grave of her husband. I realize, on looking back, how her sturdy independence and self-reliance must have sustained her during that awful time after 1930, when her husband had died and she was left virtually alone with three growing boys in a strange land. My paternal grandfather, a kindly Scot and, like all of his side of the Grieve family in Salisbury, strongly Roman Catholic, did what he could. By what arrangements I know not, we boys were kept on at St George's College, but how the fees, if any, were paid and who paid them is now beyond my ken. The background to those years sticks in my mind as, with the acute and clear perception of a child, I sensed the Anglican/Roman Catholic dichotomy between the families. Apart from grandfather Peter Grieve, I regarded them as alien to us, my mother's side – perhaps wrongly. Children can be very cruel.

During 1933, the Royal Navy cruiser HMS *Carlisle*, on the Cape Town station, sent a field gun's crew to give demonstrations while touring the big towns of South Africa and Southern Rhodesia, late in that year. I'd known nothing about it until one day I saw sailors, *real* sailors walking around Salisbury – so far from the sea. Here at last was a possible chance – why not try to join the Navy? I was only fourteen, but would be fifteen in December and, as I later discovered, the Navy would take me at that age, so long as I was fit, could pass a simple examination and had good eyesight.

With the help of a charitable institution in Salisbury, which kindly conducted correspondence with the Admiralty (via Rhodesia House in the Strand, London) and made all other arrangements, including a medical examination and, paying my fare to Southampton, I was on my way.

The three of us were destined to come to England at different times during the thirties and join up as peacetime Royal Navy regulars – myself in 1934, Geoff in 1935 and Phil in 1937. Thus we all spent the War at sea. After 1934 I had not, after all, quite shaken the dust of Africa from my feet, since among other theatres my naval service comprised the years 1935-7 on the East Indies station, which included East Africa (Mombasa, Dar-es-Salaam, Zanzibar, Mauritius and the like), on a County Class cruiser, HMS *Norfolk*, and a further two and a half years on a base ship in Freetown, Sierra Leone – HMS *Philoctetes*. By reason of its large and ineradicable population of tropical insects the ship was known inevitably as HMS 'Flock-o-Fleas'.

Joining the Navy

Early in January 1934, my mother and I found ourselves yet again at Salisbury station, my having said all goodbyes except the final one. I located my compartment on the train, standing at the old familiar platform, and discovered I would be sharing the two-bedded compartment with a large, fat, unshaven Greek chap. With a last hug and a kiss, some tears, a long blast from the whistle and an impressive cloud of steam, my second journey back to England began, this time via Eastern Rhodesia (the border town of Mutare) and Portuguese East Africa (now Mozambique) and the port of Beira. The comparatively short 24-hour rail trip was painfully slow, the train ambling along in a desultory fashion through quite thick vegetation, at times higher than the carriages and occasionally so close that one could practically reach out and touch it. I did not feel very communicative and was not keen on socializing with the Greek; I spurned the prickly pear which he kindly offered to share with me and spent most of the trip moving between compartment and observation platform at the rear of the train. In the hot, sultry atmosphere it was difficult to sleep, so I got out and spent most of the night on the observation platform. Home began to feel a long way away and I became painfully aware that I was on my own in a very large and uncertain world. The surface emotions were excitement and anticipation but I was deeply anxious, too, and wondered where this reckless foolishness might end. That particular part of it ended up alongside the SS *Llandovery Castle*, a lesser cog in the then powerful and important Union Castle Shipping Company. She was a disarmingly small passenger ship which did not look too spick and span, lying at a Beira wharf with an air of indolence.

Beginning to play the seasoned traveller, I sauntered up the rickety gangway as though this was old stuff to me, while wondering what the hell had happened to my little suitcase. Not that it could be called 'luggage' – I did not have much with me: some warm clothing for the English winter ahead, a few bits and pieces and primitive toilet gear, since I had not yet started to shave. The suitcase turned up in my cabin alright and I began to inspect my surroundings, which was very soon accomplished since it was not a very big liner, to dignify it by that name.

The vessel was as painfully slow as my railtrip down to Beira, and took a whole month to reach Southampton. A day after I boarded her she crept out of Beira and began her sedate journey along the south-east coast of Africa, calling at Lorenzo Marques (now Maputo), Durban, East London, Port Elizabeth and Cape Town. At Durban, I went ashore and swam in the sea for the first time in my life, enjoying the surf and beginning to settle my anxieties. Cape Town was magnificent – it is one of the most impressive sea approaches in the world, next to Gibraltar I would say; the looming mass of Table Mountain makes a fabulous backdrop to the town spread at its feet.

Out of Cape Town we turned north and began to wallow slowly up the Atlantic to St Helena, Ascension Island and Madeira, where little brown Portuguese boys still dived like cormorants for coins thrown into the sea from the ship. Further north – and our troubles began; it was blowing a full gale in the Bay of Biscay, that notorious delayer of ships, especially little ones, bound for England. Our captain could only turn head to wind and ride out the gale, and even then we were tossed around like a cork and the continuous racket of crockery and furniture being thrown about became very wearisome. Scheduled to arrive early in the morning, we slowly crept up Southampton water on this miserably wet winter's evening, with sleet now falling on the dirty snow on the dockside.

My grandparents had, the day before, come down from Byfleet, planning to return home in daylight after welcoming me and leaving me in the Navy's care. By the time we came alongside they had been on that dock since 6.30 that morning – now weary, damp and thoroughly depressed. Arrangements for refreshments in those days were pretty primitive, and they must have suffered. Their presence took the edge off my anxieties but I was relieved to see them into a taxi for their own journey home. My official reception was something of an augury of times ahead. A large Royal Marine Recruiting Sergeant stood on the dockside and, cupping his hands to his mouth, enquired in a stentorian bellow, 'Is Gregory Grieve on that boat?'

Standing at the guard rail, in my big Rhodesian hat, I waved like mad and yelled 'That's me – I've arrived'.

I went down the gangway and stood looking up at the military features of this enormous man, who said, 'And you are Gregory Grieve, are you?'

'Yes,' I eagerly replied.

'And you've come all the way from Southern Rhodesia to join the Royal Navy, have you?'

I proudly agreed, 'Yes.'

'You bloody fool! Get right back on that boat and go home again before it's too late.'

But it was too late, of course. He became more kindly when he said, 'We'll find you somewhere to sleep tonight and I'll pick you up in the morning for the Entrance Exam, then I'll show you where to get a train for your home in Surrey.'

My spirits sank – this wasn't the England I had fondly remembered. The black houses looked packed together like sardines and the dockside was pure discomfort. Sleet kept falling and it was bitterly cold. I followed the RM sergeant in the gloom to get a bus or tram – I cannot now recall which – and was then deposited at the grimy doorway of some sort of Sailors' Home, where I was to spend the night. 'I'll come and fetch you at eight o'clock,' he said, 'so be ready because you have to sit an entrance examination, which you *must* pass before things can go any further'.

I had a little money and bought some cigarettes, which I shared with two other chaps in a poky little dormitory with eight beds. At a low ebb, I wondered what lay in the future. All that preparation, all that travelling by train and ship – for *this*! I didn't have much capacity for philosophizing then, and could only feel miserable and very much alone. After a cold and somewhat moth-eaten night, the morning didn't offer much joy. Outside it still looked like yesterday.

Reinforced by a cup of tea and some bread and jam, I sat and stared at the examination paper – basic calculations, fractions, decimals, and a 'meaning of words' thing; it didn't give me any problems, and I looked forward to getting on that train for West Byfleet and a taste of simple home comforts. Presumably I had satisfied whoever perused my efforts, because the Navy would send for me in two or three weeks, I was told.

The RM sergeant, now strangely more benevolent, took me to the railway station, gave me a travel warrant and added some fatherly advice. 'You'll be alright,' he said, adding, 'but keep clean, act green, don't *volunteer* for anything – and don't forget pay-day.' The value of these injunctions became clearer later.

It is difficult, looking back to more than sixty years ago, to accurately portray all of one's feelings but I certainly remember some of them. It felt very grown-up to be enjoying a cigarette in a compartment all to myself and I began to buck up during that train ride to Byfleet. Youngsters were not nearly so knowledgeable or sophisticated then as now, and I wasn't very streetwise. But there was plenty to feel more cheerful about – I was going home to some comfort, I could put on airs like an old salt, the winter countryside was more appealing than the grime of Southampton docks and I had been accepted by the Navy. I anticipated a short breathing space at home before I plunged into whatever 'joining the Navy' might transpire to be. I began enjoying a kaleidoscope of 'hearts of oak' visions, of heroic poses against a backdrop of gleaming gun turrets, sailors marching about, pulling on ropes and dashing into the rigging, admirals saluting each other, triumphant lines of battleships at sea and destroyers tearing about firing torpedoes at everything.

It really was most generous of me to have gone to all this trouble and to have come all this way from Rhodesia so that the Royal Navy might enjoy my salient and important contributions to its fighting efficiency. As I walked, with my little suitcase, down Station Road, West Byfleet, to number 79 I felt seven feet tall and affected the swagger of an old sailor.

CHAPTER II

The New Entrant

On 26 February 1934, obeying the summons which had
arrived some three weeks after my homecoming, I
caught an 'up' train from Byfleet to Waterloo and boarded the
Portsmouth train. After changing at Eastleigh, I think, I
finally arrived at Gosport, across the harbour from
Portsmouth and just a short march from the Boys Seamens'
Naval Training Establishment, HMS *St Vincent* (Fig. 2), the
thirties' equivalent of its past namesake, the old hulk or
'wooden wall' which had been moored in Portsmouth
harbour and served the same purpose long ago (Fig. 3). The
nondescript gaggle of young men in cheap clothing who
dismounted from the train were in some contrast to the
rather grand station itself, the noble and classical frontage of
which consisted of a long Tuscan colonnade of fourteen bays
in Portland stone, terminating in large pavilions with round-
headed rusticated openings and parapets featuring segmental
pediments – this faded magnificence because Queen Victoria
used the station for her journeys to Osborne House on the
Isle of Wight. Years later, in 1938, because I am interested in
things architectural, I revisited the station to admire its
classical proportions – now all gone with the wind, I believe.

In the gathering dusk a naval petty officer herded the

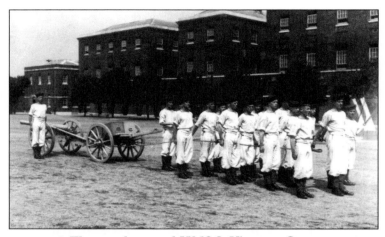

2. The parade ground HMS St Vincent, *Gosport.*

stragglers into a group beneath one of the platform lamps and began ticking off names on his clipboard, as each member of the variegated collection indicated his presence. We formed two untidy columns and marched out of the station and down the road to the arched gateway of the shore establishment – which was to be our fearsomely demanding alma mater for the coming year. 'Keep in step,' the PO kept chanting. By the gate we were ushered into a room, therein to reconfirm for higher authority that for each name on the list a living, articulate body was actually present, and were then marched around the periphery of a large parade ground, before entering a red-brick building in which we were to be quarantined for the next six weeks.

In those days the Navy drew its recruits from a wide spectrum of society – the sons of serving men, boys from the *Arethusa* training ship, waifs and strays, boys from Dr

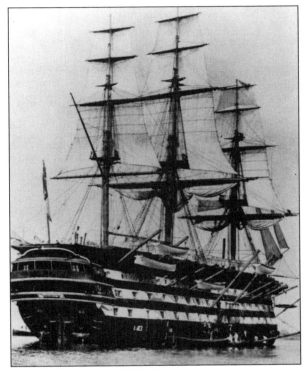

3. The original HMS St Vincent – *a 'Wooden Wall'
in Portsmouth harbour.*

Barnardo's Homes ('banana boys'), unemployed youngsters,
young men in search of clothing and regular meals and wide-
eyed boys just eager to become sailors and go to sea. Since
infection spreads like wildfire among men in close proximity
– ships and barracks – it was important to keep the
approximately thirty new entrants ('nozzers') isolated from
the main complement of 700 boys in training, until potential
infections had been given time to declare themselves. Hence

the six weeks were devoted to an initial thorough bath, dental and medical inspections, removal of all head hair, kitting out, how to look after our kit as well as our bodies, how to sew ('make and mend'), basic drills and the simple rudiments of living and working together.

Our mixed bag of some thirty boys was to comprise 98 class, of the 'Forecastle' division. Our milch-cows (or milch-oxen) for the next twelve months were to be Chief Petty Officer 'Bobby' Hales, our seamanship instructor and a truly lovable man, and Petty Officer Ben Mowlem, our gunnery instructor; an absolute bastard with an unlimited capacity for invective and wounding sarcasm. Our shepherd of the station platform turned us over to the isolation block staff, after giving us some advice: 'You'll soon shake down and find that everything that happens to you is for your own good. Do what you are told to do without question and to the best of your ability. You will live and work together as a team, so start being proud of your team.'

As ever, the first night was not a good augury. After a cup of hot cocoa and some biscuits we were given an hour or two to get to know each other and then advised to turn in – which meant getting undressed and lying on a hard horsehair mattress under a glaring electric wall-light, which remained glaring throughout yet another moth-eaten night. The plumbing of the primitive adjacent urinals was unusually noisy. Each time I woke it was to the loud and continuous twittering, gurgling noise of those bloody pipes. I still bridle at the memory of that beastly noise, now over sixty years ago.

Next day, having marched – we were getting better at it – to a long wooden hut, we were lined up at the trestle tables piled high with socks, boots, gaiters, underpants, pale yellow 'flannels' (baggy T-shirts with square necks edged in blue), blue-serge trousers and jumpers, coarse duck trousers and jumpers, blue jerseys, lanyards, blue collars with three white stripes, large black silk handkerchiefs and soft 'gibbies' (a sort of glorified beret headgear) as our instructors barked out sizes. An astonishing number of the youngsters did not know what their sizes were, no doubt not having been in a position to know those dimensions or make choices about their clothing. Each bewildered individual also received a large, strong, brown canvas kitbag. Having stuffed the contents of this horn of Cornucopia into the kitbags and deposited them in the isolation block we marched to the barber to be divested of all head hair. Extraordinary how these measure obliterated all individuality for a little while. This indignity was followed by indelible marking of the duck canvas suits and a demonstration of scrubbing them in strong soda water, to remove the dressing, soften the material and make them comfortable to wear – which they were, being cool and pleasant to the skin in hot weather. Having pitched in and scrubbed our 'ducks' I was fascinated by the monstrous spinner, a gigantic bowl which easily engulfed thirty 'ducks' and spun them virtually dry in a little more than five minutes. Added to this pile of government issue magnificence were a sort of 'donkey's breakfast' mattress and a coarse brown mattress cover, which also became paler and more comfortable with repeated washings, as we recovered, on the ranks of stark iron bedsteads in the dormitories, from the day's exertions.

We were shown how to embroider our names (lucky those with short names like 'Heap') in all clothing, also to embroider the letters 'NS' on the front of two of the 'flannels' which served as nightshirts. Woe betide any 'nozzer' (new entry) who slept in a day flannel or dressed for the day wearing a flannel he had just slept in. There was no escape from these simple and effective measures to keep us wholesome and healthy. There then followed the dreary torture of learning how to lay out one's kit for inspection. I heartily *detested* this arbitrary nonsense but got good at it in time.

For some reason I cannot recall – I was low in spirits – I began to suffer a crop of boils on the back of my neck, a succession of these revolting lesions necessitating me 'going sick' every so often and ending up in the Sick Bay getting the boils lanced and drained. A muscular Sick Bay Attendant would spray 'cocaine snow' on the place and lance the lesion to let the pus out. I suffered more from low spirits than from the boils, and used to hum to myself, over and over again, 'Happy Days Are Here Again' – *anything* to cheer myself up.

An enterprising local photographer had got permission to photograph each new entry, once we had been shown how to dress ourselves in this strange new garb. One stood against the 'ship's bell' attached to the isolation block wall and tried to look naval. My own photograph showed only a completely expressionless face, as if all individuality had been obliterated.

Then began the chivvying from pillar to post, while being exhorted to do it faster, more smartly and quicker still. The simple drilling and square-bashing, the incessant marching about, the 'left turn', 'right-turn', 'about turn', 'halt!' and 'quick march', the constant injunctions to look smart, stand up straight, hold your head up and generally being ordered about soon reduced us to thirty cloned units of respect for authority, *any* authority. The never-ending cleaning, sweeping, polishing, scrubbing, buffing up and mindless tittivating pointed us firmly in the direction of looking good at *all* times. We quickly digested that the earlier you absorbed the basics the easier life became for you. We got the sense of that classic song of the recruit: 'If it moves, salute it. If it doesn't, paint it.'

We were encouraged not to hang about.

'When you get the order to MOVE, you *fly* – and the last one gets a whistle chain across the backside.' Sometimes a 'stonachy' (a two-foot canvas sausage loosely stuffed with horsehair) did duty for the whistle chain. These instruments of persuasion were also used to clear us out of the warm showers after bitterly cold sessions on the playing fields across the road from the main gate.

'You don't walk across the parade ground, you *run*.'

'You always salute the quarterdeck' (a patch of gravel in front of the administrative building, sporting a flagpole and a white ensign).

Similar pressures were applied in the gymnasium during our first introduction to physical training. We capered up and down wall bars, learned to shin up a rope, leapt (mostly) over box horses, got expert at moving around at speed ('flying') and exercised our bodies to physical exhaustion. We didn't know it then but we were being expertly moulded into efficient fighting units, each with tremendous 'pride of ship' and eventually to make utterly dependable contributions to whatever the team might be – a gun-turret's crew, an ammunition supply group, a lookout or operator of a gunnery instrument. On reflection, we were looked after very well indeed, and I still give thanks daily for that sterling and timeless instruction in how to care for our bodies and our clothes.

As 'Boy, Second Class' were were paid 5 shillings and 3 pence a week; one shilling was given to us (with a bar of soap) and 4s and 3d put aside as compulsory savings. The accumulation was paid to us when we left to join seagoing ships at the conclusion of our training. We were also issued with a seaman's knife then. This had a large folding blade and a marlin spike. I cannot recall the pay of a 'Boy, 1st Class' but do remember that on being promoted to 'Ordinary Seaman' one's salary shot up to 8s and 9d per week. It was quite extraordinary how far a shilling would go. The return trip across the ferry to Portsmouth cost 1d and a good seat in the Queen Street cinema cost 2d. It was there I saw Fred Astaire and Ginger Rogers in *Flying Down to Rio*, in June 1934. A 1½d postage stamp was enough to write home and for 2d one could get a bar of Cadbury's milk chocolate or a packet of five 'Woodbine' cigarettes.

Our true saviour in those halcyon days was Dame Agnes Weston, a public-spirited Victorian lady who took the comfort and moral welfare of British sailors to heart. She caused to be erected, at each of the Home Ports (Portsmouth, Devonport and Chatham) a 'Dame Agnes Weston's Royal Sailors Rest' – solid imposing edifices where one could get a cup of tea, a snack or a bed, at any time of the day or night. The food was cheap and the bed cost 9d (4½p). Each bed was enclosed in a wooden cubicle, roofed over with strong wire netting to foil any would-be sodomists from climbing over the partitions and corrupting the morals of young sailors during the small hours. Since *St Vincent* boys had to be back to barracks by six o'clock we were saved from a fate worse than death. The charm of 'Aggie's', as it was affectionately known, was that if one attended a temperance meeting, a 'Sign The Pledge and Stop Your Grog' gathering, one had shelter, warmth, a sing-song and a degree of entertainment at no cost whatsoever. We sat around in this large room, with a weather eye on the wisp of steam rising from behind a screen, and the rattle of crockery, as tea was being prepared, and sang those lovely old Victorian and Edwardian ballads, like 'Pull for the Shore, Sailor, Pull for the Shore', 'The Boy Dying On the Battlefield', 'Just Break the News to Mother', 'If those Lips Could Only Speak', 'Only a Bird in a Gilded Cage' to the accompaniment of a wheezy harmonium. We were then given a cup of tea and a bun, whereupon a grey-haired 'Old Contemptible' moved in front of the seated boys and proudly drew attention to the row of medals on his chest, awarded for his years of strict temperance. We were encouraged to heed the consequences of the demon drink and exhorted to sign the pledge and renounce grog. Not that we were in any danger, since at that age we were not issued with a rum ration and could not afford alcohol, anyway. I smile at it now, but on cold winter afternoons 'Aggie's' was a warm and comfortable harbour, and I still remember those sweet old songs with much affection.

Here we might mention the irreverent nicknames of ships – the 'Tin Duck' was HMS *Iron Duke*, the 'Tiddly Quid' was HMS *Royal Sovereign* and so on. 'Aggie on Horse-back' was HMS *Weston-Super-Mare*, of course.

Our instructors, Ben Mowlem in particular, were not above the liberal use of insult and expressions of contempt and abuse. If you could not let it slide off you like water off a duck's back, you would go under. I well recall some of our class, including me, reduced to tears after a barrage of wounding insult. Classmates of sterner stuff soon had us developing psychological countermeasures, like 'And the same to you, mate' under the breath. We could never move fast enough, do things smartly enough, be efficient enough to satisfy these overbearing taskmasters. The never-ending tirade became quite monotonous. Typical examples which stick in the mind were: 'Look at you – mother's gift to a nation,' 'Ullage, that's all you are, ullage,' 'You are all useless, bloody useless,' 'My granny could do it better than that,' 'You're all as wet as piss and twice as nasty,' 'You're putting years on me, you dozy lot,' 'God help the poor United Kingdom' and 'Why should England tremble?' were some of the milder epithets. These tender words of encouragement belonged more to the parade ground than anywhere else, and did in time stimulate us to move with practised precision. The bullying had a purpose – it hardened us up, we absorbed slights with a shrug and no hard feelings, and most importantly when we had come through that horrible six weeks of isolation and for the first time marched out to join the main body of older boys on parade, we were immensely proud of ourselves and would literally have died for the honour of 98 Class, Forecastle Division. The cohesion, the glue which bound us together as shipmates, had miraculously been forged in six short weeks. I don't know what happened to Ben Mowlem and Bobby Hales – perhaps they were killed in the War or perhaps are still alive somewhere. I salute them.

Came the unforgettable day when we did march out, with the Royal Marine band playing 'Colonel Bogie', to join the main body of boys at Sunday morning 'Divisions' – a regular, full-blown weekly parade of the whole establishment. Lined up on the parade ground were 700 boys and their instructors – all wearing their uniforms with an easy confidence in the morning sunshine. I had never seen 700 white people all together in my life. There were only 64,000 whites in the whole of Rhodesia in those days and this (to me) grand array of young sailors was a most impressive sight. I began to perceive what I had joined – the Royal Navy! I got an idea of

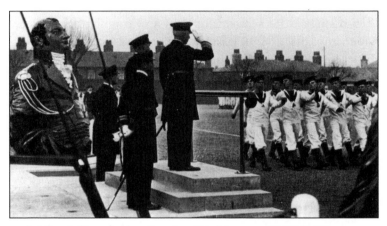

4. March Past during Sunday Divisions at HMS St Vincent.

the size of the organization of which I was now a part. Swollen with pride, I resolved to do my very best – which eventually I did, tying for first place in gunnery with a boy called Bulpitt and coming second in seamanship. We moved out of the isolation block and into the Forecastle dormitory block, aware of the superior airs of the established incumbents.

The working day started at 5.45 a.m., when we were roused out of the feathers by the bugler's 'Reveille' – he stood in the middle of the parade ground and aimed his blasted noise at the dormitory blocks. After a cup of cocoa and a hard biscuit we mustered on the parade ground at 6 a.m., in blue jerseys and duck suits in the wintertime and duck suits only in the summer.

I still recall the longing, on frosty mornings, with which we got a whiff of the Instructor Petty Officers' cigarettes, as they smoked at the edge of the parade ground before everybody dashed out and got 'fell in' for the morning's activities. We then dispersed for seamanship, physical training or gunnery, which took us to 8.30 a.m., when we had breakfast i.e. the duty 'cooks' collected food from the kitchens (the galley), served it out then washed it up. Slow eaters were discouraged; each was persuaded to 'eat it and beat it' so that washing up could be accomplished without delay.

We turned to again for boatwork, seamanship, elementary navigation – 'Rule of the Road' – knots and splices, school, 6" gun drill in the gun shed, swinging the lead (literally learning how to take soundings of the depth of water), climbing the mast ('Last one over gets a whistle chain across the backside') or marching off to Tipnor rifle range, where we learnt to handle and fire a .303 Lee Enfield rifle (First World War vintage). Markmanship was fostered and there was a tile-shooting range within the establishment. I still remember the pronounced 'kick' of the .303, even though I had used a rifle (.22) in Rhodesia.

The unlucky ones were marched down to a boatyard carrying oilskins, and were put to launching the heavy thirty-foot naval cutters, which were then pulled around 'Pompey' harbour by manhandling a cumbersome great ash oar in the biting wind. After that it was pure delight to march back to *St*

Vincent and get out of that perishing wind. There was also field-gun drill on the parade ground, and field-gun competitions – fiercely contested. Smoking was strictly forbidden and if caught you got ten days 'Jankers' – a physical punishment by way of extra drills, running around holding a rifle overhead, no shore leave, extra work and so on. You were roused an hour before the main body and were kept at it long after the main day was done. One was also marked out as a sinner by having to wear a 'nozzer's gibbie', the cap for new entries only. Yet when Bobby Hales took us sailing (in sloop rig or dipping lug cutters) or rowing around Portsmouth harbour (which we frequently did in the most bitter weather), he would produce a packet of cigarettes as soon as we were out of sight of the watchers on the wharf from whence we set out for boat instruction, then pass round the matches so that we might have a smoke. He knew damn well that no one, but *no one*, would split on him. That was a compliment of high

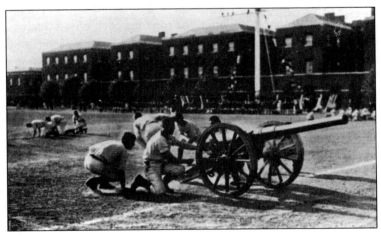

5. The field-gun competition, with the mast in the background.

order, from a truly lovable man. Since it was common knowledge that all the boys smoked while 'ashore' and in any case as soon as one got to sea there was cigarette rolling tobacco available at 2s 6d (12.5p) a lb, it wasn't such a crime.

The theory of boat-handling and small boat seamanship was initially taught at large-scale models, which were beautifully made and complete in every small detail. Every boy was able to get a good view of the six-foot models of a cutter or a whaler, with every structure, down to the smallest block and tackle, cleat or fair-lead faithfully reproduced. We learnt the rudiments of 'Going about' as opposed to 'Wearing', of 'Tacking' and 'Coming alongside in a seaway', and the arrangements of the sails and sheets (ropes) accordingly. By the time we got to the real thing in Pompey harbour we could 'go about' in a dipping-lug cutter with the best of them.

Knots and splices were taught with the boys sitting on a long bench and facing a length of rope for each boy. Attached by an eye-splice to a long wire rope which ran the length of the room, the free end provided the bit for practice. Dear old Bobby Hales walked up and down, guiding our fumbling hands and fingers as we attempted clove hitches, sheepshanks, reef knots, bowlines, eye-splices, sheet bends, rolling hitches and the like. In my day I could produce a passable 'monkey's fist' but that skill has long since sunk without trace.

Much emphasis was placed on sport, of course, although I do not recall a rugger team. Not being any good at sports which required a field or ground space (tennis, cricket, soccer etc.) I tended to shy away from them, but did shine when it came to the water. I swam and dived with more success, like most young Rhodesian boys, and dived for my port division in later years. Also, while not much of a boxer, I was, I suppose, a useful welterweight, until put in against a fearsome Scot who was clearly out to wipe me off the face of the earth; after that I left it to the enthusiasts.

One more serious skill was the necessity to swim a length of the swimming bath fully dressed in a ducksuit, thereby adding to one's chances of surviving a sinking. Instructors stood by with long poles with hooks attached, to rescue the faint-hearted and the inveterate sinkers. One boy seemed to have a propensity to make straight for the bottom. However hard he tried, beginning on the water's surface, be was soon totally beneath the surface, still going for a few strokes and heading undeniably for the bottom. I cannot remember what was done for him; the bottom just used to attract him like a magnet!

Gunnery comprised a little of practical skills with a lot of basic theory. Because we couldn't be allowed to lob 4.7", 6", 8" or 15" shells around the environs of Gosport and Portsmouth, and laying on enough of those kinds of ammunition for 700 boys would have been prohibitively expensive (besides highly dangerous to local populations), we did a fair bit of make-believe. The word 'Gunnery' conjures up the Gun Shed, a depressingly grey building containing a row of First World War 6" gun mountings, complete with breech mechanisms and all usual fittings. There was also a pile of stiff canvas aprons, spotted with what looked like blood (and *was* blood). A 6" shell weighs about 100 lb, and these had to be heaved about as in the heat of an action, slammed into and then regurgitated from the gun breeches.

We learned that *any* member of the guns crew should bellow 'STILL!' (whereupon everybody froze) when an accident looked imminent – not trauma to the flesh but an explosion. Many's the youngster who got his fingers in the way of a closing breech or got his hand in the way of a 6" shell. With Ben Mowlem yelling encouragement and obscenities at us it was not to be wondered at. We secretly despised this old-fashioned make-believe not knowing that when we got to sea and worked a real gun, there was surprisingly little difference in the basic drill. Many lives were saved by a sharp-eyed gun's crew member shouting 'STILL' and averting a high-explosive tragedy.

The gun shed stood down by a little creek of sea water, on a promontory from which one could look across to the shipbuilding slipways on the other side of the harbour. Warships were built at Portsmouth in those days and we watched the launching, in 1934, of the 7,050 ton cruiser HMS *Amphion*, later handed over to the Australian Navy as the *Perth*. The grandstand view was well worth the long wait before she slid into the water.

In the midst of life we are in death. We were all so young, so keen, so healthy and so full of go-getting competition, and on Saturday mornings a group of 'volunteers' (euphemistic word) were told off to man the great 2½-ton roller and drag it all over the parade ground, ironing out surface defects and 'divots' so that the hallowed parade ground looked good for Sunday Divisions. One of the youngsters manning the drag-ropes was the boy Talbot. We decided to get a move on and began trotting with the roller. Poor Talbot missed his footings, stumbled and fell. In no time the roller had passed over him, its great weight crushing his skull like an eggshell.

He came from South Africa, and it must have been a most melancholy task for the Forecastle Officer to telegraph and then write to his parents with the devastating news.

We completed rolling the parade ground at a walking pace and were never allowed to trot again. Talbot was given a full military funeral, which made an immense impression on us young boys. We slow-marched to the graveyard with rifles reversed, and lined up to hear the committal, and the 'Last Post' by the bugler. Shots, I cannot recall how many, were fired over the open grave and then we marched away, leaving poor Talbot far away from South Africa and in alien soil. We marched jauntily back to the training establishment to a merry march from the band, which I thought a bit much – yet we had recognized the sadness of death and life has to go on, so strike up a merry tune. It didn't mean any less respect and we still mourned him.

There were some wonderful 'Navy Weeks' in those days. Each of the home ports put on a great show to encourage recruits. The home ports were stuffed with big ships, all polished up to the nines, and simulated naval actions entertained the enormous crowds who flocked into the dockyards. In summer 1934 it seemed as though the Royal Navy was the best in the world, and the *St Vincent* boys basked in the reflected glory. We used to go ashore, mingle with the crowd in the dockyard and walk about as though we owned the place and were solely responsible for all this magnificence. HMS *Hood* ('the world's greatest warship') was in Portsmouth that year and I went aboard, acting as though this was my natural habitat – I even answered some questions from wide-eyed youngsters. Little did I know that the *Bismarck* would sink her within seven years and that I would assist in avenging the *Hood* by destroying the *Bismarck* in turn, on 27 May 1941. Small world.

Much of service life – its ethos, its humour, its characters – is just not transferable to 'civvy street'. The humour was very special and many of the characters much larger than life. The close proximity of the mess decks brought any trait more forcefully into the open, and some of the individuals with whom one lived cheek by jowl, worked with and played with stick in the mind yet. Among many was 'Splash' Akrill, who looked utterly geriatric at fifteen and even moved like a geriatric! 'Gringo' Jeans looked very Mexican and it was mildly surprising to hear a pronounced Hampshire accent coming out of his mouth. A chap called Heap also sticks in the mind (inevitably 'Uriah') – he was a neat, compact, little man who could move like lightning and was much envied because he embroidered his name in his clothes long before the rest of us. There was also 'Pig' Grower, whose physiognomy closely resembled that of a porker and who had the greed and the manners to match. He cheerfully absorbed all scorn and insults with no hard feelings whatever; I heard later he had died in action in the Mediterranean. One Commander Board, a navigation officer, had a rather Teutonic look and the back of his head was a bit flat – he was known as 'Herr Von Plank', of course. 'Robot' Dent, a great tall South African boy, moved stiffly like an automaton, as if his limbs were mechanical extensions of his body and moved by an arrangement of wires. So many faces, so many voices and characteristics which stick in the mind; many of them went down at sea yet live in my memory.

One of my happier memories of individuals concerns a

Royal Marine Sergeant Physical Training Instructor, under whose crisp commands I capered around the gymnasium at St Vincent. He was a very neat, dapper and self-contained man, whose voice and very movements were neat and incisive. I had great respect for him, since he achieved first-class results with the most uncompromising human material. He was a well-liked and very successful instructor, instilling discipline without any shouting or bombast. When, eight years later during the War, I turned up at the School of Physical Training, Pitt Street, Portsmouth to quality as a PT Instructor myself, who should be on the staff but this RM sergeant, whose teaching I had the pleasure of benefiting from all over again.

We'd heard tell of another boys' training establishment, HMS *Ganges*, at Shotley near Harwich on the east coast, but gave little thought to it since, on asking our instructors about

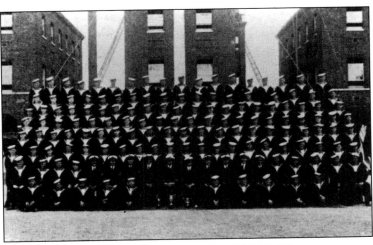

6. *The Forecastle Division 1934 HMS* St Vincent.

it, we received the comment, 'Shotley boys, Shotley bred, strong in the arm and weak in the head'. We did not, therefore, feel any sense of competitiveness.

Time To Spread One's Wings

After a year's training we were all larger, stronger, fitter and now much more use to the service. We sat academic examinations in school, and in the theory of gunnery. 'What is Rate?' 'Rate is the speed or rate of change of range, in yards per minute or feet per second.' (Got that one right, anyway.) We sat examinations in Boat Handling, Seamanship and 'Rule of the Road' – a sort of maritime Highway Code, the latter largely a matter of remembering the markings of buoys during daylight and understanding the various colours and clusters of lights at night. Some classic little jingles helped. 'Green to green, red to red, perfect safety, go ahead' referred to the port (red) and starboard (green) steaming lights when under way at sea, and indicated that when two vessels meet head on, each should turn to starboard (right) so that they present their port (left) sides to each other as they pass. Generally you keep to the right at sea i.e. opposite to road traffic in England.

Soon after completing examinations we were issued with a new blanket, a hammock and supporting ropes (nettles and clews) and a new donkey's breakfast. There followed instructions in how to 'sling' the hammock, how to make oneself comfortable (which they certainly were) and how to 'lash up and stow' in the mornings, with seven turns of rope making a large compact sausage.

'Why just seven turns, Chief?'

36

'Because six are not enough and eight are too many – and don't ask bloody silly questions.'

Early in March, 1935, 98 class went to sea – but some of us didn't, at least not immediately. After the collection of our savings (the proportion of pay kept back), the allocation of Port Divisions, issue of a seaman's knife and having packed our bags and lashed up our hammocks, we said goodbye to Ben Mowlem and Bobby Hales. Standing by our pile of baggage we noted a gaggle of new entries arriving at the isolation block – all that now seemed so long ago. Piling our belongings onto the truck which would take them to the train, we marched in a superior manner out of the main gate and down the road to Gosport station. Nine or ten of us, me included, were to go to Devonport and join HMS *Norfolk*, a County Class cruiser of some 10,000 tons, with eight 8" guns, in four turrets, eight torpedo tubes, a secondary armament of four 4" high-angle guns, anti-aircraft pom-poms and an aeroplane on a catapult. I couldn't wait to see the aeroplane, which I knew would be a Fairey IIIF biplane with a Napier in-line engine.

We were met at Devonport by a truck into which we piled our baggage and ourselves, anticipating the thrill of boarding our first seagoing ship and becoming real sailors, with the ship's name on our cap tallies (ribbons). We looked forward to something smart, bright and impressive, but saw only this great filthy, hideous mess in the middle of a dry dock. The thing wasn't even floating! Dockyard workers, not the tidiest of people, were crawling all over it, steam hammers and riveters were making a most unholy cacophony of noise and there seemed to be rust and filth everywhere. The decks were covered in a layer of dirt and iron filings, which had permeated everywhere below decks and into all living spaces (such as were not occupied by tired dockies during the day). The whole ship was a filthy, depressing, heartbreaking mess. And there was no bloody aeroplane!

Mournfully, we got our gear aboard and settled into the Boys' Mess, two decks down from the upper deck.

CHAPTER III

The East Indies

With all repairs and rehabilitation eventually completed, the messy dockies departed and we began to clear up the revolting filth. We were taught how to use a paintbrush – 'put it on from side to side and finish off from down to up' – how to scrub this and scrub that, how to polish this and burnish that, how to clean the 'corticene' covering the decks of living spaces, how to live in about a square foot to each soul, how to keep the mess decks clean and sweet. The cardinal sins were being dirty and blocking a gangway. *All* gangways had to be kept clear at *all* times. Anyone who was personally dirty was forcibly cleaned by his messmates. No hard feelings, just keep clean, that's all. Any bits of clothing left 'sculling' about were deposited in the scranbag forthwith, and could only be redeemed by surrendering a bar of soap. We gradually shook down and after about three weeks of spit and polish the dock was filled up and we moved out to tie up alongside and become a whole ship again (Fig. 7). In March 1935 we set sail for Gibraltar, Malta, Port Said, the Suez Canal and Port Suez, the Red Sea, Aden, Colombo and our principal base in Ceylon (Sri Lanka) – Trincomalee. And we now proudly carried our aeroplane.

I remember the gap between the dockside and the ship

gradually getting wider as wives, mothers, daughters and sons and babies all waved goodbye to their menfolk. We were abroad for two and a half years and those women did not see their husband again for that period. No wonder there was a certain amount of hankypanky going on in the home ports – a degree of it, anyway. It must have been pretty hard for those women to run the house, faithfully raise the kids and keep on the straight and narrow for those years. Many did just that, I know, but there was also some straying. And who could blame them. 'Let him who is without sin cast the first stone.' I know that a handful of the husbands used to go ashore and fornicate like rabbits.

Plymouth and the Hoe gradually fell behind us and disappeared below the horizon. Since we were the flagship of the East Indies station we carried an Admiral and his staff, also his flag, of course, which proclaimed our importance as we showed it around that particular parish of the British Empire. Our parish or billet included the Red Sea, the Indian

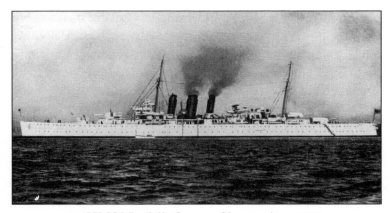

7. HMS Norfolk *County Class cruiser 1935.*

Ocean, the Persian Gulf, India, Ceylon, East Africa, the Bay of Bengal and innumerable little islands dotted around the Indian Ocean, plus Mauritius, of course.

After three days at sea Gibraltar rose above the horizon, becoming massively greater as we approached. The great awesome pile of rock, characteristically capped by its own cloud cover (the 'Levant') was a most impressive first call after leaving Plymouth. The dusty little town sprawled at its base seemed a bit of an anticlimax, yet uninformed visitors often miss the better parts of strange places. We didn't stay long, soon getting under way into the Mediterranean, with Malta another three days away. I could not forsee that the next time I trod that seaway, in 1942, it would be to enter what became known as 'Bomb Alley', and to run the gauntlet of everything the Axis powers could throw at us as we accompanied the convoys to Malta – the George Cross Island.

Malta, it seemed to me, was just hot and smelly, with those ubiquitous church bells going most of the time. The baked honey-coloured stone and arid ground was a contrast to early spring in England; it is difficult, after some sixty years, to remember anything other than that sun-baked stone.

The island was famous among sailors for its 'Strada Stretta', popularly known as 'The Gut', a sort of dowdy sunset strip of clip joints strung out along a nondescript little street. There were animated attempts at simulating sin, but for the most part it was a sad little enclave with tired 'hostesses', epitomized by the wry description 'singing and dancing, shilling a bottle' – referring to the Fosters beer which was sold there. My most salient memory of Malta in 1935 is of being 'volunteered' to join a football ground-marking party of boys, toiling in the sun to refurbish the white lines of the football pitch at Corrodina. The PO in charge of the party kindly refreshed the six of us with half a pint each of Youngers Ale, which was nectar to our parched throats. Never again, for the rest of my days, would a glass of beer taste so heavenly – probably because I didn't pay for it.

Malta is now all tourism and very good hotels, but in those days it was first and foremost an important naval base, which provided a living for very many of the inhabitants.

Port Said had its own singular odours, and while alongside a wharf there, awaiting our turn to enter the Suez Canal, we were offered everything from 'eggs and bread', and scraggy little chickens, to conjuring 'gillie-gillie' men and naughty photographs – there was a great trade in these 'feelthy pictures' which were, as ever, something of a let-down. I cannot recall anybody going ashore there – certainly we boys never got any shore leave – because we were soon on our way through the Canal, via Ismalia and the Bitter Lake to Port Suez. The Canal seemed no more than a waterway through the hot sand – with camels to look at from time to time. All I recall of the journey to Aden through the Red Sea is of a permanently-aged old able seaman advising me, 'Try not to fall overboard in the Red Sea – it's full of sharks.'

Aden, the commercial capital of the Republic of Yemen, is built on two peninsulas, each with a high volcanic headland of largely barren rock baking in the sun. It has been a trading centre since Roman times and was taken by the British in 1839. It became an important coaling station and transhipment point after the opening of the Suez Canal in 1869. Its importance to Britain was manifest in the presence not only of the Royal Navy ships of the East Indies station but also two RAF stations, Khormaksar and Shaykh Uthman – the latter airfield comes into my story later. In 1937 Aden became a Crown Colony and subsequently was the scene of fighting between nationalist groups. When Italy invaded Abyssinia (Ethiopia) in 1935, strategic considerations dictated the presence of a British naval force at the southern entrance to the Red Sea. Thus it was that we found ourselves back at Aden on a semi-permanent basis, at least during the latter part of 1935, including Christmas, and the early weeks of 1936. After our initial call we gratefully sailed out of that baking suntrap and began to enjoy sea breezes again as we made for our 'home' bases of Colombo and Trincomalee in Ceylon (Sri Lanka).

Here I must describe a characteristic of the Indian Ocean which I never observed in other waters, and that is of a completely flat calm and a glassy smoothness of the sea surface – so much so that when the surface is seen to be disturbed by a ripple ahead, it transpires to be caused by a turtle. Clouds and the odd rain squall are seen marching along the horizon, but around the ship the air is so still that funnel smoke appears to hang above the ship and move with it. I recall several occasions when there seemed not a breath of air, or movement, in the world, except our sultry and soporific progress across the surface of the ocean. A far cry from 'Winter North Atlantic'. Then on other days there was a bit of a sea running, and porpoises would come tearing around, shooting out of the water in a graceful arc and playing around the bows. There were flying fish, too, of course, literally flying for their lives as they were pursued by marine predators. I saw more whales in the South Atlantic, en passant between Cape Town and Southampton, than I ever did in the Indian Ocean but perhaps I wasn't looking in the right direction at the right time.

The extraordinary thing about Ceylon is that one smells it a whole day before one sees it. The spices are in the air and on the wind as one approaches that beautiful island. I find it hard to equate my memories of that gentle Singhalese people sixty years ago and the recent pitiless and fearsome bloodshed between Government forces and the Tamil Tigers. More sophisticated people with more sophisticated weapons and more sophisticated discontents. Even the savagery has gone up-market.

After arriving at Colombo we lay in dock for a little while, incongruously surrounded by coconut palms. I'm not too sure of my chronology at this point, but do not feel I need trouble the Admiralty for precise facts of what came before or after which – in any case it is not really important. I think it was about then (April 1935) that the *Norfolk* departed on an Indian Ocean and East Africa cruise. We pointed our bows south-west and made for the first of a handful of islands we visited, including Diego Garcia, of the Chagos Archipelago. I recall the obligatory coconut palm trees, the white sand and the low-lying foreshore. The first night there was quite magical, with a fat, pale yellow moon shining a path across the water and the gentle south-east trade wind blowing – the memory of it is still acute. The only European inhabitant of one of the islands – was it Diego Garcia? – was a Portuguese lighthouse keeper, whose request for reading material we could meet with out-of-date newspapers and old magazines (the *Tatler*, the *Sphere*, *Titbits*, and *Humorist*, the *Passing Show* and *Country Life*), many of which have long since sunk without trace. He welcomed this magnificence with open arms, and expressed his gratitude by sending out several boatloads of pineapples, yams, coconuts, bananas and other tropical fruits, together with several woven baskets of every kind of fresh fish, all piled on the deck. It took some considerable time to distribute this amplitude to the messes and the cold store room.

Other islands we showed the flag to were Mauritius, of course – that cosmopolitan, polyglot place – and Agalega, a mere spit of sand covered with coconut palms and fringed with casuarinas. Also Mahé in the Seychelles, Farquar Island, Astove Island, Aldabra and then west to East Africa, calling at Dar-es-Salaam, Zanzibar and Mombasa.

Mauritius, previously uninhabited until discovered by the Portuguese in the 16th century, is a volcanic mass thrust up from the depths of the Indian Ocean a little north of the Tropic of Capricorn. It is about the size of an English county and was first Dutch and then French. In the thirties it was still a British Crown Colony, having been taken by conquest, and after 158 years as such became independent. It has been a republic since 1992. The main crop is sugar, with tourism now added, and the island is still 'French' in so many ways, not least the place names e.g. Port Louis, the capital, and Curepipe, Vacoas and Quatre Bournes. Although the official languages are English and French, the majority of the population are of Indian descent, with European, African and mixed minorities.

Behind Port Louis rises Le Pouce, or The Thumb, like a fist with the thumb erect. During half the year the south-east trade winds blow upon the island, enveloping the heights in cloud and mist and producing dazzling rainbows. The clouds steadily build up during the day and at Curepipe, for example, in the middle of the island, they regularly deposit showers at about four o'clock in the afternoon. Parts of the island are quite mountainous, rising abruptly and spectacularly from green, palm-fringed foreshores to their carved pinnacles which catch the morning sun. They are not very high, only a little over 2,500 feet, and carry no mantle of snow, only the ever-present plumes of cloud. Their naked sides expose flanks of basalt a thousand feet high, with long-tailed tropical birds wheeling about them like blown pieces of paper. In the north rises the Pieter Both Mountain, a sheer 2,700 feet pinnacle and visible like a church spire over much of the island.

The polyglot nature of Mauritius is manifest in the multi-ethnic inhabitants, their styles of dress and their places of worship, e.g. the Jumma Mosque in Port Louis (Fig. 8). I don't know what degree of socializing between the races exists there now, but before the War what was known as 'the colour bar' increased the complexities and difficulties of life, and social circles remained rigidly enclosed. Life was lived in private and behind closed doors – an affair of clubs. Not that this troubled the sailors of HMS *Norfolk*; the heavy and claustrophobic atmosphere of social taboos was plain enough but as very temporary visitors there was no call, and certainly little opportunity, to become embroiled in something which was above our heads, anyway. Also, servicemen soon become adept at doing in Rome what the Romans do. The advent of airborne tourism and multiple hotels has probably made a lot of difference but I am writing of sixty years ago.

Although not always guided by my nose, it seemed to me that Port Louis, in those days anyway, was a somewhat ramshackle and odourous place, gently stewing in its own juice. Yet parts of the island are very beautiful, and I would

46

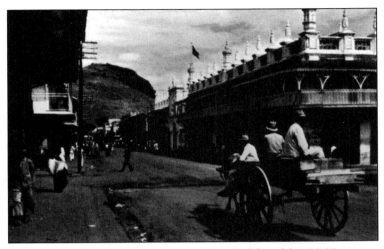

8. The Jumma mosque, Port Louis, Mauritius 1947
(F.D. Ommanney).

have preferred to get to know it better before sailing away. Boy seamen do not have the money or the time ashore to go exploring in foreign parts. We visited Mauritius just once more during our stint out there, and that was in the spring of 1937, on our way to home and beauty after completing our commission on the East Indies Station. I went ashore with a chum and we visited the local racecourse, mingling with the crowd and becoming enchanted with two lissom French girls whose eyes promised the earth but did not deliver. They were quite captivating, reducing us to willing slaves.

Apart from Diego Garcia (if I *have* got that right) and Mauritius, my memory cannot distinguish between the five other islands or archipelagos we visited. They were each like the others. I do recall that the boys were not allowed ashore at Mahé, in the Seychelles; a good thing, perhaps, since there was a noticeable increase in the incidence of 'social diseases' in the ship's company after leaving those beguiling islands. Sailors who contracted venereal disease ashore had to live segregated in a special mess, apart from the main body of men and using only special cutlery and utensils. Inevitably, the mess was known as 'Rose Cottage'. Today one reads, with wry amusement, enticing advertisements for this, that or the other holiday, at considerable expense, in the places one sweated in with discomfort, all those years ago.

We turned north-west and made for the East African coast, our first call being Dar-es-Salaam, memorable for its dazzling white beaches, which were quite blinding in the sun until one got used to it. A series of picnics were arranged for the boys' usually at one beach or another, and very happy occasions they were. Dar-es-Salaam was so clean and beautiful.

While there the Roman Catholic boys (of which I was nominally one) were invited to an early morning Mass at the local cathedral, to be followed by a breakfast, laid on by the hospitable nuns of a local convent. I *think* they were French, and they leant over backwards to put on a real show. There was nothing special about the Mass, other than the soaring proportions of the cathedral, but the breakfast was the eye-opener of a lifetime. Some twenty people, guests and incumbents, sat at a long, wide table which had been beautifully set with silver cruets and ornate dishes fit for the pomp and circumstance of a royal feast. The flowers, the cutlery, the napery and the place settings were quite magnificent, complemented by the dozen or so native attendants in crisp white suits, grinning from ear to ear with evident enjoyment of the occasion and showing rows of teeth as white as the beaches; they were having as much fun as we

were. After the fairly basic food we'd been used to, we made
utter pigs of ourselves, of course, wading with gusto into the
fruit juices, the bacon, eggs, sausages and kidneys, pancakes,
fruit, piles of toast and hot coffee from the most ornate jug as
big as a small water-butt, it seemed. I really don't know what
we had done to deserve such magnificence; their hospitality
was manifestly heartfelt and I warm to it to this day. We had
nothing to offer in return but to say 'thank you' dozens of
times and to enthusiastically hug the nuns. We were returned
to the ship in a spankingly-smart 'Admiral's Barge' type of
harbour conveyance. There were interesting reminiscences,
by some of the older citizens, of the exploits of the German
cruiser *Emden*, which operated, at times, out of Dar-es-
Salaam as a commerce raider. She covered immense
distances and was a thorn in the side of the Allied powers for
some time during the First World War. She overreached
herself by attacking the cable station at Cocos Island in the
Indian Ocean, at the same time as the first Australian-New
Zealand troop convoy was passing on its way to Egypt, and
she was destroyed by HMAS *Sydney* on 9 November 1915.

After Dar-es-Salaam, Zanzibar was a bit of a let-down, and
all I can recall of it was the incongruous sight of an ample
and stark naked negress doing an imitation of the cancan,
accompanied by a spirited rendering of Offenbach on a
mouth organ. Whether it was a brothel or a clip-joint I cannot
now remember, but it could not have been up to much since
a boy seaman's pay did not purchase luxuries.

While we lay alongside at Kilindini, Mombasa, several of
the older seamen got a few days' leave, and returned with tall
tales of a trip up-country to Nairobi, in a motor car with a
souped-up aero engine, driven in a maniacal kind of way by a

bit of a show-off, over not very well-maintained roads. The hair-raising trip to Nairobi was capped by meeting up with the driver's chums, and a drinking session of truly Bacchanalian proportions, which they had to join, of course. They seemed relieved to get back to the comparative peace and quiet of the ship.

We pointed ourselves north-east again and made for Colombo, there for half the ship's company to be sent up to a rest camp in the hills, among the misty tea plantations of Ceylon.

Living below decks in a man o' war is a little different to enjoying the well-ventilated comfort of the Colombo Galle Face Hotel, for example. Although the mess decks of the County Class cruisers were much roomier than some of the older cruisers of that era, they were not really suitable living spaces for men existing cheek-by-jowl in the hot, steamy climate of Colombo at sea level. For some decades before my time out there, it was the custom for ships' companies to be given several weeks' leave during the hottest and most uncomfortable months, and to enjoy a breather in a camp up in the hills. We entrained at Colombo, almost alongside the ship, at dusk so that the journey to the camp would be during the dark hours; we then slowly chuntered up and up into the heights of the tea plantations. There are some awesome gorges and precipitous slopes to wonder at from the railway carriages, and the night journey was a precaution against everybody crowding to one side to look and thus capsizing the narrow-gauge train. The climate at that height is very much like that of England, and the cool mists and moderate breezes so very welcome after the muggy, itchy heat of Colombo. The camp, at Diyatalawa, in the Kandy/Nuwara

Eliya area of the high centre of the island, consisted of a series of dormitories or airy, long huts, open to the night air and, if my recollection can be relied upon, with a mosquito net to each bed. There was absolutely nothing to do but enjoy the climate and occupy oneself with walks, sport and whatever diversions we could cook up. We were woken in the morning by the Singhalese attendants bringing us a cup of tea, and all cooking, serving and washing up were in their hands – we did not have to touch a utensil or a tea cloth.

Altogether it was the life of Riley for the denizens of HMS *Norfolk*'s lower deck. The tea planters could not have been more hospitable – they even laid on dozens of old golf clubs, and some old balls and gave us the run of their golf course. We were not too careful of the nicely kept greens, alas, which suffered a degree of mayhem. The kind planters raised not an eyebrow, since labour was cheap and grass grew like wildfire. There was also provided a 'Chase the Greasy Pig' event, when some 250 sailors lined the edges of a hockey pitch and tried to grasp a well-greased piglet after it was released from the centre of the pitch. Also a fancy dress occasion, the variety of costumes bearing witness again to the infinite capacity of the British sailor to rise to the occasion. Parades and musters and the like were kept to the absolute minimum and every man jack of the crew thoroughly enjoyed a good rest for several weeks. In the absence of women, men make their own diversions, and the standard of some of the ship's concerts, 'Sod's Opera', was very high indeed. There is a goldmine of talent on the lower deck of a naval ship, and the uninhibited nature of the setting allows some truly great performances. I can still hear the bawdy 'Ringa Ranga Roo' being belted out from the makeshift stage.

The weeks passed much too quickly, and came the time to pack up and get the little narrow-gauge train once more, this time downhill from Diyatalawa to the coast. Back again at Colombo, in much better shape and with the prospect of some not too demanding sea-time, we sailed south, then east then north, skirting the island as we made our way to the naval base of Trincomalee. 'Trinco' is just about the finest natural harbour in the world. It is an extensive and well-protected anchorage, becoming of vital strategic importance during seaborne operations against the Japanese in the latter part of the War.

In my day there was little there but some superb swimming, lots of palm trees, a herd of working elephants and a 'canteen' – the euphemistic term for a long palm-thatched hut which sold beer at reasonable prices but not much else. There were some oil-storage tanks and probably much other of 'furniture and fittings' befitting a naval base but I don't recall noticing anything other than I have described. The base was comprehensively upgraded during the War and must now look most unlike those carefree, innocent days of 1935.

There was wonderful swimming at 'Trinco' – the countryside by the shore was like a tropical Garden of Eden, a brown-skinned tropical paradise. One could see the sandy bottom of the little bay through the limpid clear water; and there was no need for bathing trunks. Swimming there in the crystal sea was much more than just a 'skinny dip' – it felt like sloughing off the tired, grubby skin of civilization and going back to nature. . .

While there with the other ships on the station, we held a 'Fleet Regatta', one of the events being the Boy Seamens'

Cutter Race, during which several young men and myself rowed like maniacs, trying to manhandle a great, heavy ash oar. I forget who crossed the line first.

★   ★   ★

HMS *Norfolk*'s movements during 1935-7 could broadly be grouped as the East African cruise (already mentioned), the Persian Gulf cruise, including calls at Karachi and Bombay, the South India cruise and the Bay of Bengal cruise, including calls at Calcutta and Rangoon. The normal sequence of 'showing the flag' here, there and everywhere was dislocated to a degree by the necessity to remain at Aden for many months in late 1935 and early 1936, because of the Abyssinian conflict.

From Trincomalee we returned to Colombo, before departing for the Persian Gulf, our first port of call being Muscat, after which we visited Bushire and then sailed up the Shatt al-Arab water way to Abadan and Basra. Abadan was developed from a small village after the discovery of oil in 1908. It is now a major port and oil-refining centre with petro-chemical industries. Basra, an oil port of Iraq is one of only two shipping outlets to the Gulf. The two pervasive recollections of our time in the Gulf were (i) the sand, the heat and the flies, and (ii) the whiff of the oil refinery at Abadan. One just could not escape that miasma of fuel oil. Other memories are of the great hospitality of the British community in Abadan: they laid on a most entertaining concert for us. It was during 1935, at one of the Gulf ports, that we said farewell to our Fairey IIIF biplane and hoisted on board a brand new Supermarine Walrus amphibian flying boat. I was captivated by the sight of this glamorous silver flying machine, lying secured to a buoy near the ship and seen through a porthole near my bed in the Sick Bay. I enjoyed a mild bout of malaria and an interesting new aeroplane at the same time.

During a second visit to 'Trinco' during 1936, the pilot of the Walrus – then known as the 'Pusser's Spitfire' and later, during the War, as the 'Shagbat' – offered flights to any of the ship's company who would like to have a go. I jumped at the

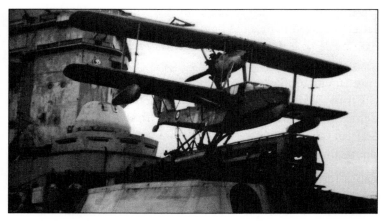

9. Supermarine Walrus aircraft and bridge structure,
HMS Rodney.

chance, and enjoyed several landings and take-offs from the smooth water of the enormous anchorage. I still have a vivid mental image of the emerald-green shallows of the harbour and the lovely sands, seen from 5,000 feet. We also carried a Walrus on HMS *Rodney* (Fig. 9).

Heading down the Gulf we called at Kuwait and then Bahrein. I was struck by the extent of the shallows – the ship had to anchor well out from the shore and motor boat journeys from ship to jetty seemed to take for ever.

After calling at Karachi, and undertaking some primitive 'combined operations' with a Baluchistan regiment, which involved landing a field gun from a cutter and other bits of military hanky-panky, we sailed for Bombay, the fabled 'Gateway to India'. The brothels in Bombay are, or were, in Grant Road, and on the urgent recommendation of a chum who could vouch for the excellence of the service provided, I visited this one particular establishment and enjoyed the expert and understanding attentions of a maternally-minded prostitute. Inexperienced young men are full of eager but ham-fisted, fumbling ignorance and need a great deal of careful teaching. Initially, they do not understand that a woman's skin is like a musical instrument, and that while the sudden clumsy grab just makes for discord and turn-off, the caress of gentle handling, begun slowly and courteously, can produce the most beautiful music. I began learning in Bombay, and to this day give thanks for that patient lady who taught me and who was selling her body that she might give her daughter a good education. She gave me one, too.

If my memory is sound, it was after Bombay that we returned once more to Colombo and then sailed to Aden, there to stay, in that baking oven, for weeks and weeks and weeks, even unto Christmas 1935 and after. Despite the uncomfortable heat, we doggedly conducted Christmas with all the usual paraphernalia of decorations and gluttony – there were decorations, Christmas dinner, plum pudding, mince pies, and rum for the older members of the ship's company. No wonder we got an Empire together!

Earlier I mentioned two RAF stations at Aden, Khormaksa and Shaykh Uthman, the latter being equipped with a squadron of Hawker Hart biplanes. These fast and manoeuvrable two-seater aircraft were the RAF's standard light bomber during the first half of the thirties and were beautiful aeroplanes. They have been described as 'the most technically and strategically significant bomber design of the ten years following World War I' and nearly 1,000 of them were built. The reason for mentioning these facts is that the *Norfolk*, together with other RN and RNZN ships then at Aden (*Diomede* and *Effingham*) often went to sea for gunnery practice, night shoots and general maneouvres. By invitation the RAF chaps used to come along for the ride, and a day or two at sea must have been a very welcome change from the dust and heat of their sun-baked aerodromes and living quarters. In return, they invited the ship's companies for an early morning flight over the desert. This was manna from heaven for me, since it was the first time I flew – and in what an aristocratic aeroplane! I got my name on the list at once and have often puzzled why so few responded to this exciting invitation. Early in the morning the ship's boat deposited us at the landing stage, there to be picked up by the RAF truck which took us out to Shaykh airfield, where the Hawker Harts stood glistening in the earlier morning sun – a thrilling prospect. We were strapped into the parachute harnesses after some hair-raisingly rudimentary instruction how to pull the ripcord if we had to bail out, and were then assisted into the aeroplanes – I was practically wetting myself with excitement. Without delay the engine roared into life and we taxied to one end of the airfield, turned toward the far end and then belted down the desert field in a great cloud of dust. I

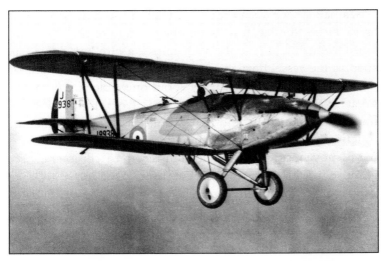

10. The RAF Hawker Hart biplane of the 1930s (RAF Museum).

realized there were no more bumps – we were flying, and it was quite beautiful!

After the heat at ground level the cool air was a delight, as the eight planes soared and wheeled in formation over the brown desert floor under our wings. Everything was enchanting, the sun on the wings, the whistle of the wind in the flying wires, the almost solid slipstream, and the hardly detectable movements of the control surfaces as we banked and turned. We were up there for about an hour, and as requested the pilot of the machine I was in obligingly side-slipped into land because I wanted to see what it felt like. After that magnificence, a simple breakfast and into the truck to go back to the landing stage and get the boat back to the *Norfolk*. For weeks afterwards, the ship felt very mundane and earthbound.

Seamail (there wasn't much airmail in those days) used to arrive every Sunday, usually on one or other of the Peninsula and Orient liners (the 'P 'n O' ships), a gun being fired as soon as the vessel hove in sight around Steamer Point, one of the harbour headlands, usually about one o'clock. There was great excitement on Sundays. Mail from home was an important happening and men would gaze at the headland, practically willing the ship to get a move on as the minute hand moved to one o'clock, and eager to catch the first glimpse of its bows appearing round the point. Other happenings, which helped to relieve the monotony of lying at Aden in the enervating heat, were cutter sailing trips and picnics. We would load corned-beef sandwiches, baskets of oranges and 'fannies' (a type of mess-deck drink container) of lime juice into the cutter lying alongside or tethered to the boom, paddle away from the ship's side to catch the wind, and then hoist the sails, proceeding out of the harbour and a little way along the coast until we spotted a likely beach. After beaching the cutter we'd swim in the shallows, keeping a lookout for sharks, stuff ourselves with corned beef and oranges, sleep and sunbathe, sailing back to the ship at the end of the day. In all of my fifteen years in the Navy, I was seasick only once, and that was in a sloop-rig cutter in Aden harbour. There wasn't even a decent sea running – it took months to live down the shame of it

I can recall little else of note – Aden is a monotonous place – other than a sea trip to Port Sudan, halfway up the Gulf, the purpose of which escaped me, and one to Port Suez which was more interesting. We stayed for a day or two and a trip by taxi to Cairo was laid on for the boys. It was arranged for us to visit the Cairo museum – mummies and Pharoahs galore – and the Spinx and the Pyramids, which in those days was a camel ride outside Cairo. There were not enough camels to go round; I and a few others ended up with diminutive Arab donkeys, upon whose backs it seemed an imposition to sit. I would have felt morally more comfortable walking, which one could practically do with the tiny donkey between one's legs. The whole trip was culturally dutiful rather than enjoyable – a taste of life in the more naughty bits of Cairo would have been more popular. We were just itching to get into adult forms of sin – which we did soon enough, of course, mainly in Calcutta and Rangoon. During the taxi ride we noted by the roadside the odd dead tree, and sitting in its branches a scraggy collection of vultures.

Early in 1936 the international situation became less fraught and we thankfully left Aden and made again for Colombo, and 'Trinco'. After some more comfortable 'sitting about', we set sail on a cruise around the southern tip of India, the beautiful Kerala. Travel brochures today describe it as a paradise – it was more so then, an unspoiled Garden of Eden. We called at Cochin, and the beguiling ports of Trivandrum and Tuticorin. There was an air of unspoiled innocence, a childlike trust in the essential goodness of life, which was so much to the fore in those beautiful places.

Recollection of the sleepy beauty of palm trees, soft white sand and opalescent sea is easy, because one saw so much of it, but what has stayed in the mind more than anything else is the feeling that one was a child again and that it was an unpolluted, unspoilt world. I believe this still characterizes the people of Kerala. Time seemed to have stood still then, a bucolic tropical paradise like 'Trinco', and utterly different from the urban materialism of Bombay, Calcutta or Rangoon.

There is nothing else to describe because nothing else happened! One just enjoyed the beauty of the place.

Perhaps this is the point to dwell on a factor which is probably part of the twilight of the British Empire. F.D. Ommanney, in *The Shoals of Capricorn* (1952) mentions that one of the many reasons why the British lost India was that, while yielding more and more to the Indians politically, they persisted in holding them at arm's length socially. The more they yielded politically the more socially up-market they became. I quote:

> I have often wondered whether the mass of people really care at all that much about political liberty or know what to do with it when they get it. It is an elusive thing and they usually immediately lose it. But nowadays, with the spread of Western education, they do care deeply about social equality, personal liberty and decency in everyday life. That is why self-government is everywhere preferred to good government. To always be subordinate and inferior in one's own country is held to be intolerable. The awakening of Asia is not so much a determination to get rid of the oppressive, or even of the extortionate foreigner, for in truth he was not often either, as a determination to get rid at all costs of the contemptuous and snooty foreigner, the foreigner who shouts at you, shuts doors in your face, who bars you from his clubs and his home. Not that you want to belong to his clubs or be invited to enter his home, but you do not like being barred from them. This social barrier is, I believe, largely a feminine creation, invented by women.

During the middle months of 1936 we spent more time at Trincomalee and Colombo. My memory is vague about that period. We began the Bay of Bengal cruise late in that year

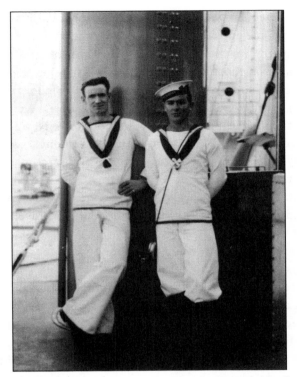

11. HMS Norfolk *in Calcutta 1936 – author as a bugle boy.*

and by December were in Calcutta (Fig. 11). The 11th was my birthday and on achieving eighteen I was allowed to stay ashore until 11 p.m. – big deal!

The junction of the Indian subcontinent and Burma is one of the most densely populated areas in the world. It is no more than a vast delta, a low-lying alluvial plain, cut by a network of rivers, canals, swamps and marshes. Calcutta, the largest city in India and the port capital of West Bengal, is close to the border with Bangladesh and lies on the Hooghly river in the Ganges delta. A certain proportion of its 11 million people appears to live mostly on the streets.

Navigating up the Hooghly river to Calcutta and tying up alongside is a most demanding exercise for the river pilots, because the configuration of the subdelta is inconstant and there are currents which can quickly take charge of a carelessly handled ship. The city is a polyglot mixture of over-population spilling out onto the pavements, wretched poverty, cheek by jowl with the pomp and circumstance of military splendour and old Indian Army units like the Bengal Lancers, that famous cavalry regiment. We viewed a parade of the regiment on Calcutta Racecourse, and a brave, stirring sight it was.

These are the impressions of a young man, sixty years ago. Perhaps things are different now.

There was a great deal of entertaining on board. Having spread awnings over the quarterdeck, scrubbed the deck and polished brass-work to within an inch of its life, we prepared the setting for a series of cocktail parties and dances. In the cool of the evening the ship looked like a fairyland, with soft, strategically placed lighting adding to the glamour of the scene, glinting off the burnished muzzles of the guns and enhancing the womens' dresses and the medals and uniforms. A succession of important guests came up the gangway as the Royal Marine band played selections from Strauss and Gilbert and Sullivan in the background. During the day the ship was thrown open to visitors, and I was intrigued to note a young Sub Lieutenant eagerly escorting, around the bridge, a girl in a flowery dress. She was from the brothel in Cariah Road and I had spent a session with her two days before. I'd tried to take my time and not be too urgent about things but was instructed to 'get on with it'. No doubt an optimum level of production had to be maintained. I hope she made the Sub Lieutenant happy.

On our departure from Calcutta, a small flotilla of little boats, carrying young ladies, followed us for a mile or two down the Hooghly river – apparently we had made an impression.

Not so, to my knowledge, in Rangoon (now Yangon), where we arrived early in the New Year. Strangely, I have no recollection of Christmas 1936.

Rangoon lies on a river of the same name, whose delta is part of the greater delta of the Irrawaddy. It became the capital of Burma in 1885 and has always had a large Indian and Chinese population. A more peaceful country in the thirties, the war with Japan and subsequent internecine strife have contributed to its economic troubles. Since post-war independence, the exports of rice, teak oil and rubber have declined. I recall the magnificence of the Sule Pagoda – 2,000 years old – but little else of Rangoon. My recollections are that we socialized much more with the Army at Mingladon barracks, on the periphery of Rangoon, than we did with the indigenous population. Perhaps we were recovering from the fleshpots of Calcutta. One cameo remains in my mind – the sight of a twin-engined KLM monoplane (a 'Fokker'?) skimming across the delta and outlined against the setting sun. The idea of aeroplane travel was in the air in those days and one instinctively knew that one was looking at a lusty infant which would grow strong in the years to come.

When we crossed the Bay of Bengal again, making for our 'home' base of 'Trinco', we went east and added some southing – 'Left hand down a bit'... and we were beginning to think of the long haul back to England, to home and beauty.

As ever, we smelt Ceylon the day before we got there. Its spicy scent was in the air and on the wind, the north-west monsoon. It was almost like coming home to see 'Trinco' again, and a pleasure to go ashore and enjoy the bucolic tranquillity of the place. No fleshpots, no sin, only sun, sand, swimming, cool beer and thoughts of home. Several weeks were taken up with sea exercises, night shoots and another impromptu regatta involving the ship's company only, before we left Trinco for the last time and did the right-hand circuit of the island to get to Colombo again. Eventually we turned our bows out of Colombo and began the long roundabout journey to England and Plymouth, via Mauritius, Astove Island, Aden, Port Suez, the Canal, Port Said, Malta, Gibraltar, the Bay of Biscay and the English Channel. I have mentioned earlier the two lissom young French girls who captivated my chum and I on our second visit to Mauritius, and there is no need to talk of it again but at Astove Island, another spit of sand covered with coconut palms, 700 miles south-west of the Seychelles in the Aldabra group, there was (like Diego Garcia) a manager who had been there for years, with only the occasional spell of leave in the Seychelles. Also, Ommanney described the stout, jolly manager of Peros Banhos, in the Chagos archipelago, who'd been sitting on his atoll for sixteen years, occasionally visiting Mauritius for a holiday. 'All of these people remained spry and alert and interested in life and none of them had taken to drink ... for anybody with an active mind it must have been durance vile.' There is little to do, other than sit and gaze at the white beaches and the turquoise sea through the coconut palms –

with the tiresome presence of Creole-style red snapper on every menu. Of the Seychelles, a travel writer has recently remarked that with its rain-forest-covered peaks, its stretches of coral sand and its well-positioned modern hotels, Mahé can be pretty seductive. 'My advice, however, is to get out fast.' Sand so pure and fine, sea so blue that you gaze at it with bewilderment approaching nausea ... too much pleasure can be a dangerous thing. We left Astove island and headed north, and as the baking rocks of Aden appeared ahead the prevailing mood was 'This time we are not staying but passing through, DV' – which we happily did. We went rolling home, ticking off the succession of hot, sticky places as we left them behind, our bows pointing west, west and ever west, until we rounded Gibraltar and turned north for the Bay of Biscay.

Some may have regretted leaving behind the scented East but I was glad to be shot of it. We approached Gibraltar on a bright and sparkling, breezy morning and the Rock looked magnificent and proud. The fresh salt air felt so *European* – odorous places and sultry miasmas were now in the past. There, on the far side of the Rock and through the Straits of Gibraltar, was the Atlantic, the lovely European Atlantic. It was a truly festive moment on a jewel of a day. The whole world and all the waves seemed to be leaping up to touch the sun. I felt hugely potent, with the sun tearing at my spine and the whole creation leaping with the joy of life. The clean breeze blew away all the grubbiness and boredom – even the ship itself appeared to quiver with expectant trembling ...

The green hills of Devon welcomed the *Norfolk* as she came home to Plymouth on an early June morning in 1937. I was shaving near a bathroom porthole as we passed

Eddystone lighthouse, and there between us and the light-house was the black dorsal fin of a shark – probably an amiable basking shark. That little cameo sticks in the mind to this day.

Within the hour we were alongside in Devonport Dockyard and wives and sweethearts were streaming eagerly up the gangway – some carrying babies. Don't know whose the babies were – we'd been away for over two years.

One half of the ship's company went off on a month's leave immediately, the other half (me included) remaining to see the ship into dry dock for attention to rudder and screws, scraping of underwater surfaces and application of anti-fouling paint. We spent a month in the uncomfortable circumstances of being in dry dock – no water supply on board therefore no toilets or bathrooms available. There were noisome dockside facilities provided but this was no better, so as far as washing and shaving were concerned, than filling a bucket on the dockside and bringing it back to perform one's ablutions in familiar surroundings.

We had come full circle – the ship soon began to resemble the very same filthy state in which we had first confronted it in March 1935!

Soon my turn came to go on leave – and I never saw the *Norfolk* again, since I returned to HMS *Drake*, the RN Barracks at Devonport.

CHAPTER IV

The Last of the Thirties

In July 1937, Able Seaman Grieve stepped off the *Norfolk* for the last time and made for North Road Station, Plymouth, to catch the Great Western Railway express to Paddington. I crossed London to Waterloo and was soon on the next train to Byfleet, with the prospect of seeing my mother and brother Phil again after three years. While I was abroad they had come to England again to live with her parents. Some years after the death of my father she had married again but it was not entirely smooth water, it seemed. I never knew quite why, or any of the details, but there seemed reason enough for her to uproot her Rhodesian connections and come home to England.

It was a lovely and excited welcome, with everybody talking at once. She looked well and I was pleased to see that. Brother Phil had grown, of course, and wanted to hear all about the Navy. Me having rolled up with a deep tan, a sailor's uniform and full of tall tales nothing would do but for him to join up as soon as my leave was finished. He too, ended up at *St Vincent* – he said he was proud to see his brother's name on the 'Roll of Honour' board in the Drill Shed. It was customary to inscribe names of those who came top in Gunnery and/or Seamanship. Yet he well surpassed my efforts since he was selected for promotion to Leading Boy, which was more than I ever was.

The great thing about Phil is his enthusiasm. Once he becomes enthusiastic about anything, he goes like a bomb, and I can well visualize the enthusiasm with which he threw himself into *everything* the Navy expected him to be good at. He went on, during 22 years in the Service, to get his commission and retire in 1959 as a Lieutenant. He went back to the large horizons and the subtropical climate of Southern Africa, which he loved. Both he and his wife became actively involved in countering the terrorist activity in Rhodesia. For his pains he got a terrorist assegai through his knee, and now walks with a pronounced 'gimp' to one side. He tries to put it away as the rolling gait of an old sailor, but my belief is that he is referring to sea time on the Gosport Ferry. In truth, when he was on HMS *Cumberland*, another County Class cruiser, early during the War, the ship chalked up the greatest sea mileage of all, much of it in the South Atlantic. He was of the company of ships waiting for the *Graf Spee* to emerge from Montevideo, and they had the gratification of sailing past the scuttled and burning ruin of the German ship. Why, I wonder, do Germans seem to take so much pride in scuttling their own ships? They appear to take pride in having scuttled the *Bismarck* – if they actually did (see later).

The beauty of being in Byfleet for a month in the summer of 1937, and having a few modest funds, was that one could get a train up the line to Weybridge, the home of a flying club as well as Vickers and the Brooklands track, and walk across the bridge over the track to the flying club HQ. One could get a flip in a Puss Moth (five minutes for 5/-) and I spent a fair bit of money on flights. I once splashed out for a ten-minute flight and persuaded the pilot to do some stunting. We looped the loop three times and I gloried in it. On the last loop I thought I'd test the straps holding me in the cockpit, and as we reached the height of the loop I just folded my arms and let the straps take the weight – which they happily did. I must have been mad; a shaky strap could have sent me plummeting to the ground. Those lovely flights, in real biplanes, were worth every penny to me. The next time I flew in a De Havilland Moth was in Perth, Western Australia, in 1994, and the pilot was my fellow physiotherapist, Brian Edwards.

Woking was just one stop down the line and going to the cinema there with my mother was a real joy. We saw Gary Cooper in *The Plainsman* and *The General Died at Dawn*, Claude Rains in *The Invisible Man* and Ronald Colman in *The Lost Horizon*. Another treat was to go shopping together at Bentall's in Kingston, to be followed by a visit to the pictures and tea. She had decided during my leave to go back to her second husband and did so in August of that year. She never returned to England again. We did not know she had less than ten years to live – she was only forty-two.

At the end of my leave I returned to Plymouth and entered the gloomy Naval barracks – HMS *Drake* (Fig. 12). It seemed an ominous and forbidding place and I was to be detailed off as a 'Guard' bugler (having learnt my expertise on HMS *Norfolk*) which meant that one sounded off the morning and evening routine calls – 'Reveille' and the like – and also performed at official functions and funerals. For example, I was detailed to sound the 'Still' – a form of salute – when the ship bringing home the body of Ramsey MacDonald came alongside the Devonport Dockyard in 1937. We lived in the

Guardroom by the main gate (Fig. 13) and did not have to sling our hammocks in the gaunt dormitories of the main living blocks. We enjoyed special titbits from the galley (cookhouse) and it was easy although illegal to slip out to the shops if we wanted anything immediately. I learnt to play Mah Jong in the Guardroom and whiled away many an hour playing that fascinating game.

My interest in girls far exceeded my capacity to pay for expensive courting, but much could be achieved during summer evening walks along Plymouth Hoe, since there were innumerable little corners with garden seats, away from curious eyes, and enticing little walkways and paths, which I got to know like an old hand. There were failures, of course, and one indignant young lady split my lip with a stinging right-hander. Nevertheless, I enjoyed several passing entanglements. On one occasion all I could afford were sixpenny seats, in a Union Street cinema, and shamefully accepted a small loan from the girl so that we could sit in slightly more upmarket seats.

Life became more real and earnest when I was detailed off to join a Seaman Gunners Course, a three-month period of training in Gunnery which fitted one for handling *any* piece of ordnance, from a .45 Webley to a 15" gun turret. This included a trip to Chatham and gun-turret training on HMS *Marshal Soult*, a shallow-draft vessel which mounted a 15" turret for shore bombardment. These vessels were called 'monitors' and only drew a few feet of water, the purpose being to get as close inshore as possible and then belt away at opposing land forces. They were named after the first of its kind, the *Monitor*, an ironclad of the American Civil War. We got so used to the turret drill that instead of shouting 'left

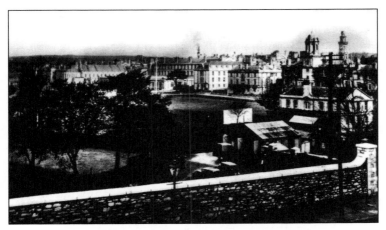

12. The Royal Naval Barracks, Devonport.

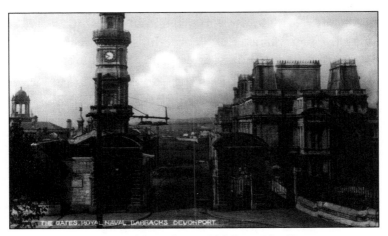

13. Main gate and gatehouse RN Barracks, Devonport.

gun ready' or 'right gun loaded' or whatever it was, one would shout 'left gun fish and chips' or 'right gun Aggie Weston's' – although everyone knew precisely what was going on, of course.

I went ashore at Gillingham, next door to Chatham, and got involved with a most attractive little maid of Kent. In fact, I nearly plighted by troth, and am glad now that I didn't – but it was a close call. Perhaps it was fortunate for her, too. Who knows? On completion of the course, on which I gained an 85 per cent mark in the finals, I was drafted to HMS *Mackay*, a 1914-18 destroyer which had been upgraded. This was more like it – thank God it was not a big ship. Destroyer life is the best there is. Everybody knows everybody else, and there is a camaraderie, a ship's spirit, which is too often lacking in big cruisers, aircraft carriers and battleships. We spent the first few days enthusiastically redecorating the ship from top to bottom and I looked forward to a happy time. Which was short-lived – after just ten days on the *Mackay* an order was received for me to join a draft for HMS *Rodney*, a great lumping monster of a battleship with three triple 16" gun turrets, a secondary armament of six double 6" gun turrets and four 4.7" high-angle anti-aircraft guns, famous for producing an ear-splitting 'crack' which was far worse than the shattering roar of the 16" guns (Fig. 14).

Misery indeed – my heart sank with forboding as we marched down to the dockyard once more, halting alongside this massive wall of steel which transpired to be the ship's side. I could see it all – it would take forever to find one's way around the ship, there would be 'crushers' (ship's police) galore and it would be just like a floating barracks. Which it was. This was in September 1938 and I served on that great

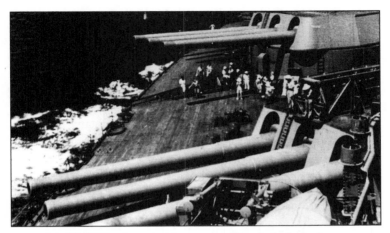

14. HMS Rodney, *with turrets trained abaft the beam.*

lumbering monster for some three and a half years, until March 1942. It's complement was about 1,500 men, if my memory serves, and I never did get to know all of them. I kept encountering strangers!

Shortly after I joined the *Rodney* we sailed round to Portsmouth to go into dry dock – the only berth of that kind available to us just then. It was enjoyable being in Pompey again. I visited my old alma mater *St Vincent* and felt very superior, with an East Indies commission under my belt and my boys' training days some three and a half years in the distant past. It was a strange, fraught time and manifest that the 'war clouds were gathering'. Hitler's territorial transgressions, each after a renouncement of any more, were becoming too blatant to ignore. Civilians were digging trenches in their gardens and there was a general air of preparation for Armageddon. All naval personnel had to carry gas masks whilst ashore, and we all felt a bit ridiculous going to pubs and dances ('shilling hops') lugging these bulky unromantic appliances. I went to a dance at Southsea and got interested in a young lady, who wanted to know 'What are you carrying that thing for?' 'We have to, I'm afraid' I replied. It wasn't very conducive to amatory progress and that promising episode fizzled out.

Then Sir Neville Chamberlain went to Germany to parley with Hitler and on 29 September stepped out of his plane at Northolt and waved a bit of paper, announcing to the assembled company 'Peace in our time'. It wasn't, but we were given a vital year in which to build more Spitfires and really gird our loins for what we knew was coming. It felt much better to face the thing squarely.

And here I must confess to a shameful misdemeanour. On joining the *Rodney* my Action Station was to be part of the team handling the right-hand gun of 'A' turret. Since there was little to do during working hours in dock, another chap and myself cleaned out all the grease cup of the gun and put back the caps of the cups, to be refilled next day, but we forgot to fill them again with grease. This mental aberration was discovered a week later by the turret Chief. I was henceforth banished from the turret and relegated to the high-angle ammunition supply chain, which meant that during 'Action Stations' I would be well down in the bowels of the ship, in the shell magazine – not an attractive place to be since if there is any danger of fire or flash reaching the magazines they are immediately flooded, all hands in that space being drowned like rats. I paid quite dearly for my lack of application. Within two years, I'd be slaving like a maniac in the 4.7 magazine for some seven hours, with short breaks, off the coast of Norway in 1940.

For some reason I know not, I have no recollection whatsoever of Christmas 1939 or New Year. My first memories of that year concern the spring manoeuvres of the combined Home and Mediterranean Fleets. Home Fleet ships were dark grey and Med Fleet ships light grey. The two fleets met at sea off Gibraltar and what a sight that was! Never to be seen again in such numbers and in such grandeur. The whole horizon, from left to right, was just ships – battleships, battlecruisers, aircraft carriers, cruisers and destroyers, the light grey coming out of the Straits of Gibraltar and the dark grey coming down from the English home ports.

After a short spell at Gibraltar the fleets put to sea for extended exercises, target practice as day shoots and night shoots, and fleet manoeuvres. We had a real gutful of being closed up at Action Stations night after night. There were also general drills, like manhandling collision mats, streaming paravanes (anti-mine procedures), oiling from tankers at sea and any other muscle-flogging routines My Lords of the Admiralty could cook up. The result of the various simulated battle actions were subject to the most stringent analysis and a great deal was learned from them. Imaginary ships had crept up on us and blown us out of the water or we had blown them to Kingdom Come. Submarines had registered unsuspecting carriers in their sights and unsuspecting submarines had been detected and theoretically blown to bits with theoretically well-placed patterns of depth charges. It was all taken very seriously and did indeed improve our performance at what we were really for. With the combined Fleet manoeuvres completed, the ships gathered at Gibraltar for socializing in each others' wardrooms and messdecks, runs ashore, cinema shows and concert parties on board, then the Fleet Regatta, Fleet Athletics and Boxing Championships.

I met brother Geoff in Gibraltar then and we had a good run ashore. I'd only seen him once before since he joined the Navy and that was in Plymouth in 1937. I saw him only once again, also in Plymouth, before he left the Navy in 1947 and went back to Rhodesia, this time working in administration of copper mining in the North. He died of a massive heart attack in the early seventies. We had not been very close and it gave me a deep happiness to have come much closer to him, via a series of long letters between us, than I ever thought I would. We three brothers had perforce been widely separated in various ships and meetings were rare. I saw more of Phil after we had left the Service than I ever did during our service. I recall one meeting in Hval Fjord, Reykjavik during late 1941, when his corvette and my battleship were stationed in that cold, desolate place waiting for the *Tirpitz* to come out of her Norwegian fjord hiding place. I got a boat to go across and visit him, and it was a happy moment. He is now living in Spain with his second wife and enjoying his grandchildren, who are scattered about the globe. We, too, have become much closer and that has given me much happiness. When one's time is nearly up, family become important.

After the nose-to-the-grindstone work of manoeuvres and then the fierce competition of regattas and boxing championships the ships departed on the customary annual flag-showing visits to the Mediterranean resorts, Madeira and British resorts like Blackpool, Weymouth, Torquay and the like. The *Rodney*'s first call was Madeira and a chum and I had a high old time visiting the wine cellars and tasting the

76

distinctive Madeira wines – sercial, bual, bastardo and malmsey. Bastardo is no longer produced, I understand. Pity.

We also had a high old time visiting the bordellos. Portuguese establishments of this nature seem to have a charisma which is missing from those of other nationalities. For a very reasonable number of escudos, I forget how many, one could enjoy the lady of one's choice, and I became mildly enamoured of a tall, willowy girl who wore glasses and seemed to take a shine to me. She also seemed to enjoy intercourse with her shoes on. My chum (Mac) had also found a transitory soulmate, and going down to the bordello whenever we went ashore became, for the 2-3 weeks we were there, like catching the 8.35 to work every morning. Mac had this unfortunate passion for stringed musical instruments and one had only to mention the words 'guitar' or 'ukelele' and he would get a glazed look and start talking of how he would like to have studied these instruments at the Royal Academy of Music.

We were returning to the ship one evening, with a fair bit of time to spare, and we had just enough of the wherewithal to finance a short visit to our lady companions. By agreement we changed direction and made for our alma mater. Unfortunately, we passed a music shop with various stringed instruments in the window, including a ukelele priced at just about the amount we had to pay for a visit to our ladies. Mac changed his mind and wanted to spend all of the cash we had on this damned instrument. We had something of an argument and decided to toss for it. Tails, he won – so no bordello but at least we (or *he*) had a ukelele. On the way to the boat which would take us out to the anchorage at Funchal, he began plucking at the strings – which broke. So there we were – no ladies and no ukelele either! I kept a photograph of the lady as a keepsake for some years, until it went down with a whole lot of other chaps' possessions as we scrambled to get off a sinking troopship four years later.

Having briefly mentioned Fleet manoeuvres, this may be a good time to discuss the handling characteristics of the *Rodney*. During our time at sea I did several tricks (spells of duty) at the wheel of the ship. She was an absolute pig to steer, as her manoeuvring capability left much to be desired. She answered the wheel with reluctance, and one had to develop the patience to put on a few degrees of course alteration or correction and then wait for the bows to come round as she slowly answered the helm (Fig. 15). The unusual appearance of the *Rodney* and her sister ship *Nelson*, with the entire main armament forward and the super-structure aft (Fig. 16), has been mentioned as a cause of their difficulties of handling, but opinions differ. It has been said: 'They were indeed slow to answer to the helm, and tended to turn into the wind, being difficult to hold on course when any sort of wind was blowing. At less than 8 knots the manoeuvring capabilities of these vessels is affected, and the high superstructure aft causes difficulties in handling them until experience has been gained.' The tall, eight-sided, enclosed superstructure had its advantages, though. The tower-type bridge that was such a distinctive feature of *Rodney* and *Nelson* was a considerable improvement on the open-platform, tier-type bridge, and was incorporated in all new construction and reconstruction. The arrangement was peculiarly British and no equivalent was seen in foreign battleships. It provided solid support for the main armament directors and gave much improved accommodation for

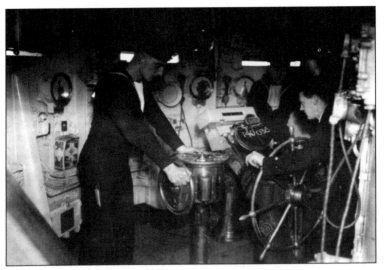

15. *The wheelhouse of HMS* Rodney.

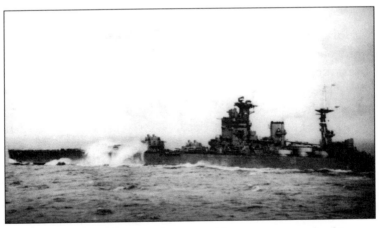

16. *HMS* Rodney *under way, with gun turrets trained to starboard.*

various bridge functions, besides providing better protection from the weather and thus improving the comfort of bridge personnel.

We left Madeira for Plymouth and after a short stay went east along the southern coast and anchored off Weymouth. Going ashore from our anchorage entailed a drifter coming alongside to accommodate the number of men who wished to sample the delights. A chum and I decided to go for a lay on the beach and a swim. It was Whit Monday 1939 and a truly English hot summer day. We spent the whole of the time on the beach, wearing only swimming trunks. Despite having been 'raised', as the Americans say, in Rhodesia and having served two commissions in the tropics, a total of five years, the only time I have been badly sunburned was that day. The reason is not far to seek – we got talking to a couple of girls sitting on the sand, and just stayed and talked, and talked, and talked. It began to dawn on me that there was something very special about one of them – Barbara Stevenson. We went off for a swim and came back to talk to the girls. Then they went back to their hotel for lunch and on their return we continued talking to them. Barbara got a little concerned about the amount of sun we were absorbing and generously emptied her bottle of Skol (is it still made, I wonder?) over my skin – I still have that bottle, sixty years on. I wanted to know a great deal more about this girl and we made a date to meet again at a local dance. That evening, on returning to the ship, I began to be very ill and was admitted to the Sick Bay for treatment. Plainly, I'd overdone the sunbathing. I was not able to keep the date and did not see Barbara again until the summer of 1940. Luckily I'd got her address and we began a correspondence which continued throughout the War, while she was being bombed to hell in London (Streatham SW16) and I was 'pounding the briny' (at sea) chasing Germans. I knew by then that she was very special and nothing would do but for me to try and persuade her to spend the rest of her days with me. Which she eventually did some six years later. We saw each other again during my short leave in 1940 and again in 1942, when we visited Kew Gardens and I proposed. We met again in 1943, after I had qualified as a Physical Training Instructor, and then not again until March 1945 when the war in Europe was nearly at an end. We married in the July of that year, and had forty-six happy years together – but that is another story.

It was a strange time – we knew instinctively that we were living out the end of an era, a twilight, and that profound changes, and total dislocation even unto Armageddon, loomed in the distance. Everybody was now aware of the massive scale of German rearming, and there was an ominous tinge to the news of yet another aggressive territorial audacity by Hitler. The British Hawker and Supermarine aircraft factories were turning out Hurricanes and Spitfires, respectively, as hard as they could go. The *Rodney* began to spend more time at Scapa Flow, our northern base, in company with other naval units. Gas masks were being turned out in prodigious numbers and there were signs on all sides that we should prepare for something big and frightening. There was talk of rationing of food and the evacuation of children, of building shelters in gardens. It was unwise to plan too far ahead, to go too far away for holidays; it was circumspect to draw together, to make a 'circle of wagons, with women and children in the centre'. Preparation for something real, immediate and nasty had begun – both mentally and physically. The *Rodney* did not come south again until March 1942, when we entered dry dock at Liverpool. We heard all kinds of rumours, that Wrens were taking over administration in the home ports, even to handing out the weekly pay packets. Later on we had the agony of knowing of the bombing of homes and cities, of no reply to letters because the house had been turned to rubble and its occupants blown to bits – the agony of knowing that Plymouth and Portsmouth and Chatham were suffering their own more terrible Guernica – by the same Stukas, Heinkels and Dorniers which did their practising during the Spanish Civil War.

A disadvantage of the *Rodney* and the *Nelson* was their lack of speed. The *Rodney* could barely touch 22 knots and was plainly in need of a thorough cleaning of her fouled hull plating. Accordingly, a short time before war was declared on 3 September the ship came south as far as Rosyth and went into dry dock there for her bottom to be scraped – by us – as a matter of urgency. It was all done at frantic speed and every man jack of the ship's crew (even unto cooks, carpenters, painters and sick bay 'tiffies') fisted hold of a scraper and scraped like hell. We started standing on rafts, so that even as water was being pumped out of the dock we began scraping off the barnacles and accumulated fouling which so reduced our speed, and we continued scraping as the lowering water level exposed more and more of the plating. Then we were right under the ship, an eerie experience, and scraping over our heads. As we scraped, antifouling paint was applied, everybody working through that first night. Within minutes of completion of the painting, the floodgates were opened a degree and water began filling the dock – the *Rodney*'s bottom was respectably covered with water again. To the best of my recollection, the whole operation was completed the next day, and we'd gained a vital knot or two of speed. We sailed north again; entering Scapa Flow to join the rest of the Home Fleet units there.

'Scapa' in winter is desolation unto desolation, but in summer and autumn it can be the most delightful place. Calm summer evenings are truly beautiful there, with the lovely evening light on the muted browns and greens of the low hills. On calm evenings a faint 'plop' indicates a seal playing around the anchor chain, and at night the 'Aurora Borealis' (the Northern Lights) are very beautiful. There was little other than beer at the canteen and football on Flotta in those days, and my chum Mac and I used to walk across the fields to find a farmhouse and get a 'tea'. The Orcadians were the most hospitable and gentle people, and we would be welcomed to share new fresh bread, farm butter, bacon and eggs (as much as we could eat for 1/6d (7.5p). I recall talking to a young daughter – she must have been thirteen or fourteen – by the fireside as our 'tea' was being prepared and asking her if she did not ever want to go to the mainland. She thought for a bit, then replied, 'I think I'll bide where I'm at.' That young girl had far more philosophy than I did, I reckon.

Sea time seemed cut to a minimum (saving fuel?) as we approached that fateful day on 3 September 1939, when, if Hitler had not halted his invasion of Poland, it was to be war. An ultimatum was issued from Downing Street: 'Unless an assurance is given that you will withdraw your troops from Poland it will be war between us.' Then we heard the measured tones of Neville Chamberlain '... I have to tell you that no such assurance has been received, and we are therefore at war with Germany.' we were at sea at the time and I was on the bridge as a meteorological assistant – I used to decode the weather data and plot it on the area charts. I expected to see periscopes of German submarines popping up all over the place. The Met officer turned to me and said, 'Grieve, I think you'd better go below and get your gas mask.' I remember thinking, 'What a silly idea. Who wants a gas mask in the middle of the bloody ocean?'

At home, the Prime Minister had barely finished speaking to the nation on the morning of 3 September when air-raid sirens began wailing across London. The false alarm sent hundreds of thousands scurrying for the nearest shelter. Preparations were already under way, with fat barrage balloons lazily floating overhead to deter enemy planes, and London railway stations crowded with reservists and volunteers entraining for their units, the soldiers mingling with parents saying goodbye to tearful children being evacuated. In countless suburban gardens, householders piled the earth onto corrugated 'Anderson' shelters.

On that day began the Royal Navy's total involvement, without let-up, for the duration – six and a half years – of the War. To have lost the war at sea would mean losing the War. To appreciate the total involvement of the Royal Navy and the RAF Coastal Command, it is necessary to briefly consider the background to the Battle of the Atlantic. Several factors governed the nature and the intensity of the titanic struggle by Allied forces to keep open the Atlantic sea lanes to Britain, and by German U-boats and surface raiders to prevent seaborne supplies reaching the UK. Among these were:

- the comprehensively prepared U-boat force and its high morale
- the submarine 'wolf pack' concept
- the effect of the 'pocket battleships'
- the chronic shortage of British convoy escort vessels
- the only moderate effectiveness of sonar detection (Asdic) methods
- lack of appreciation, in the inter-war years, of night action by submarines
- ignorance of the anti-submarine potential of aircraft.

The U-boat force. After the Armistice in November 1918, the Treaty of Versailles (June 1919) placed strict limits on the German armed forces, including a total ban on submarines, but the defeat of 1918 did not interrupt German interest in the submarine or its use as a weapon. Even as the First World War flotillas were being surrendered a great store of accumulated knowledge was being applied to lay the foundation of a submarine fleet for the next war, however and whenever it might come. In short, the Battle of the Atlantic grew out of its 1914-18 predecessor, and the boats and crews of the First World War were effectively parents to those of the Second World War. And the same men did it. The human embodiment of this continuity was Karl Doenitz, a submarine commander at the end of the First World War and chief of the submarine service between the wars and throughout the Second.

During the thirties, Winston Churchill had warned again and again of the menace of German rearmament, and it was during those years that the *Kriegmarine*'s plans began gathering pace and Germany started producing weapons again.

In September of 1935, Captain Karl Doenitz took command of a flotilla of nine new U-boats. The 250-ton craft were small and cramped, so much so that their crews referred to them as 'dugout canoes'. The men were soon plunged Into a rigorous training programme which fostered enthusiasm to rebuild Germany's elite force, the U-boat arm. This Weddigen flotilla, named like all flotillas after First World War U-boat aces, became the instrument with which Doenitz applied his theories of submarine warfare, improved his techniques and provided training for new officers and men. The Weddigen flotilla became a floating classroom. Training was so rigorous that each new crew and their commander had to complete sixty-six surface, and sixty-six submerged, attacks before being promoted to using torpedoes. The elite force soon developed a mystique, attracting the best talent among officers and men. There was fierce competition to get into the *Kriegsmarine* and standards were remarkably high. The numbers of officers and men applying to join the U-boat arm exceeded by far the numbers of places available.

The 'wolf-pack' concept. The *Kriegsmarine* proposed a method to overcome the disadvantage suffered by U-boat captains whose underwater speed was often lower than that of the convoy ships. If groups of submarines were disposed in a chain on the surface, where their speed exceeded that of the merchant ships, they could identify the approach of convoys across a wide swathe of ocean, be directed in concentration against one and inflict mass sinking by overwhelming the escort vessels. After acquiring the French Atlantic ports, these tactics were facilitated.

<u>Effect of pocket battleships and other surface raiders.</u>
German rearmament was not confined to submarines, as
surface ships (torpedo boats and cruisers) were added during
the twenties. Included in the 1928 estimates were plans for
the first of three Panzerschiffe – pocket battleships with six
11" guns in two triple turrets, medium armour and high
speed. It was plain that these were intended as commerce
raiders – confirming the *Kriegsmarine*'s preoccupation, from
above and below the surface, with destruction of the
seaborne supply of material to the enemy – Britain. Perhaps
this is not quite fair, since Ireland & Gibbons (1996) state
that the plan of operation was that the *Bismarck* would attack
the battleship escorting the convoys while the *Prinz Eugen*
would attack the merchantmen, although this is not to say the
bigger of the two ships would not also attack merchant ships,
if it had dealt with the escort warship(s). So obsessed was the
German High Command with dislocating seaborne supplies
to the UK that they recruited their two greatest battleships,
the *Bismarck* and the *Tirpitz* (of 53,546 metric tons each) as
commerce raiders. The consequences of these two powerful
battleships escaping into the Atlantic and attacking convoys
did not bear thinking about.

<u>Shortage of escort vessels.</u> With extraordinary disregard for
the bitter lessons of 1917, it was at first believed unnecessary
to put merchant ships in convoy, and parsimonious govern-
ments accordingly blocked funds for escort vessels. That is,
until 1938, when the Admiralty reversed its earlier views and
advocated the institution of a convoy system. Yet the
Government were *still* cutting escort vessel production from
naval expenditure. Only in the spring of 1939 were funds

authorized for a crash programme of fifty-six 'off-the-shelf' corvettes.

Sonar submarine detection. In 1936, the Admiralty's faith in the sonar detection of submarines was enshrined in a memo: '... the submarine should never again present us with the problems ... of 1917'. It was also believed that one destroyer could do the work of a flotilla, and accordingly new destroyers and convoy escort vessels were deleted from the navel estimates. Far from being the 'all-seeing underwater eye', the Asdic apparatus was comparatively inefficient, being limited to ranges of often less than a mile and to searching with a narrow beam at a fixed angle. The sound impulses from the transmitter only operated at low speeds and were severely affected by rough water and high speeds. Also, it needs a very experienced operator to distinguish between the echo from a submarine and those of different layers of water, fish, whales, wrecks and the seabed.

Night action. The Admiralty believed that submarines would or could not operate at night, this despite that U-boats often successfully attacked at night in the final stages of the First World War. All submarine exercises, between the wars, had to cease at night. Yet many an Allied merchant ship went down at night, as surfaced U-boats got inside the convoy because they were not detected on the surface in darkness. The Admiralty's view was all the more incomprehensible since Asdic is, or was, ineffective against U-boats on the surface.

Aircraft. The potential of anti-submarine patrol by aircraft had also been virtually ignored, probably because aircraft alone had not sunk any U-boats during the First World War. Yet there was plenty of evidence that they had a useful role to play in forcing submarines to remain submerged, thus markedly reducing their effectiveness. Coastal Command started the War with 300 fewer aircraft than it had in 1918, and these were unsuitable for patrolling long distances over sea; and their crews were untrained in anti-submarine operations.

The magnitude of the Navy's long drawn out effort is not well appreciated even now, sixty years on. The First Sea Lord himself wrote: 'If we lose the war at sea we have lost the War,' and the Navy dare not lose. The stark fact is that the Navy was fully engaged, without respite, in daily sea operations from the first day to the last day of a six-and-a-half years' war. Not for the Royal Navy the interludes between battles and campaigns enjoyed by the British Army, or the more than three years of preparations enjoyed by the Royal Air Force before it launched its mass bomber offensive in 1943. The Allied invasion of Europe in June 1944 – the greatest and most complex combined operation in history – had been planned by Admiral Sir Bernard Ramsey, and the Western Front was reopened just four years to the month after the French collapse had closed it in 1940. Notwithstanding the comparatively small number of troops who were dropped by parachute or landed by gliders, it was the Royal Navy which successfully delivered the invasion complex onto the beaches of Europe. Yet this day might easily never have happened, so close to exhaustion and collapse did British sea power come in the years 1939-43. Churchill said that the only thing which really frightened him during the whole of the War was the German U-boat campaign.

The Navy was desperately over-stretched by having to fight three separate enemies – Germany, Italy and Japan – across the worldwide spread of the British Empire. Correlli Barnett mentions that it was the Navy which had to pick up the bill for Britain's predicament at the outset of the War – too much to defend and too little to defend it with.

It suffered grievous losses in the service of Britain's Mediterranean and Middle East strategies which, although the only option after the collapse of France and the Western Front in 1940, proved enormously costly in resources for comparatively minor results.

The losses at the battle for Crete, for example, included:

SUNK: Cruisers *Calcutta*, *Fiji* and *Gloucester*; Destroyers *Greyhound*, *Imperial*, *Kashmir* and *Kelly*; DAMAGED: Battleships *Valiant* and *Warspite*; Aircraft Carrier *Formidable*; Cruisers *Ajax*, *Naiad*, *Orion*, *Perth*; Destroyers *Hereward*, *Kelvin* and *Napier*. Keegan remarks that 'When the tally was taken, the Battle of Crete, though less shocking than its effects on British morale than the future loss of the *Prince of Wales* and the *Repulse* was to prove, was reckoned the costliest of any British naval engagement of the Second World War.'

A monthly carnage in the Atlantic until 1943, the losses at Crete and in the Mediterranean generally, the monumental battles in the Pacific and the Indian Ocean, the Russian convoys and the disaster of convoy PQ17 are salient reminders of the broad canvas upon which the Merchant Navy and the Royal Navy shed their blood and treasure in such huge proportions, for six and a half years, without let-up.

The first months of the War were representative of all wars – mind-numbing boredom and utter weariness for 97.5 per cent of the time, interspersed with short, sharp periods of furious explosive action and stark terror.

As part of the Second Battle Squadron, comprising also the *Nelson, Royal Oak, Royal Sovereign* and *Ramilles* under the flag of Admiral Sir Charles Forbes, the *Rodney*'s first areas of operations were the North Sea and the North Atlantic. For most of those early months of the War we worked out of Scapa Flow in the Orkney Islands, patrolling the North Sea, intercepting enemy shipping and searching for German surface raiders, particularly the *Gneisenau* (we confronted her just once, in March 1941, when she rapidly made off into the gathering dusk). The *Rodney* also shepherded a valuable cargo of iron ore from Norway and delivered it safely to the UK.

After the brilliant attack, by submarine U-47, on the night of 14 October, when the U-boat penetrated the boom defence of Scapa Flow and sank the *Royal Oak* with heavy loss of life, the Fleet operated out of Loch Ewe, and Greenock, on the west coast. *Rodney* and other heavy units were away from Scapa, searching for a strong German surface force, led by the *Gneisenau*, which had made a probing sortie into the North Sea.

In late September, the British submarine *Spearfish* had been badly damaged by depth charges off the Horns Reef and was left unable to dive; she had to limp across the North Sea on the surface. A cruiser squadron and a destroyer flotilla were despatched to shepherd her home, and Admiral Forbes directed the heavy units (*Rodney, Nelson, Hood, Renown* and the carrier *Ark Royal*) to cover the operation. In the forenoon of 26 September, the British ships were spotted by a German flying boat, which called down nine Heinkel 111s and four Junkers 88s, carrying 1,000 and 500 lb bombs respectively.

The groups of aircraft attacked separately and in a most uncoordinated way. The Heinkels had no success but the Ju 88s were more aggressive, dive-bombing the *Ark Royal* and achieving a near miss. Also, one bomb glanced off the *Hood*'s quarter and disappeared into the sea. The German propaganda machine made much of the 'destruction' of the *Ark Royal*, repeatedly broadcasting 'Where is the *Ark Royal*?' The performance of both the bombers and the Fleet AA gunnery was poor. Both sides learned important lessons.

Considering the state she was in when war was declared, the *Rodney* did well to hold up as long as she did. Completed in 1927, she was in need of a refit when war was declared, and it exacted a heavy toll, causing her early retirement from active service. Her operational life came to an end in November 1944, when if fit for it she would have gone out to the Pacific theatre and joined the action there. She finished her days as the static flagship of the Commander Home Fleet, at Scapa Flow. She was finally broken up in 1948. Nevertheless, she gave a very good account of herself, the variety and extent of which is summed up on pp. 160–2. In November 1939 the Fleet proceeded to sea to try and intercept the *Scharnhorst* and *Gneisenau*, which had just confronted and sunk the gallant AMC (armed merchant cruiser) *Rawalpindi*. The German ships avoided detection and reached Wilhelmshaven on the 27th undamaged except for a battering from the heavy weather. *Rodney* and *Nelson* continued to search for two days in the vile weather, the *Rodney* developing serious rudder problems. She had to return to Liverpool and dry dock for stiffening of the fore part of the rudder. The same attention was given to her sister ship, the *Nelson*.

CHAPTER V

The North Atlantic and the
Norwegian Campaign

The necessity for rudder repairs allowed us time for a short leave during Christmas 1939. And so came the end of the thirties decade which had ushered in profound changes of attitude and philosophy in so many people. Recognition of the potential of air travel, fostered by the flights of the Americans Wiley Post and Amelia Earhardt, the New Zealander Jean Batten, our own Sir Alan Cobham, Amy and Jim Mollison, Bert Hinkler and Clouston and others had made people more globally aware. The advent of the Abyssinian War in 1935 increased that awakening sense of now being part of one indivisible world. The early transatlantic clipper flights via the Azores, and the flying boat journeys to the Middle and Far East, by a series of hops, added to the dwindling of isolationist innocence. For myself, the world began turning upside down on the death of my father in 1930, and in comparison to my childish settled outlook before that year, it has remained upside down. I still feel as a child of the thirties, so I suppose I haven't 'grown up'. I look back with regret as well as nostalgia for the way we were then; there was a kind of social glue and a climate of mutual trust which bound us all together. Sadly, we have lost it. We are all predators now, feeding off each other ... and devil take the hindmost.

But on with my tale, which is that the early forties, in my recollection, seem taken up almost entirely with monotonous plodding forwards and backwards across the Atlantic to Halifax, Novia Scotia, with convoys. Once or twice we took nineteen days to get across, moving at the speed of the slowest ship in the convoy. Of all the miserable, dangerous and depressing environments on this earth, 'Winter North Atlantic' takes some beating. Little wonder that 'WNA' is enshrined in the Plimsoll Line on the side of seagoing ships. The loading of cargoes had to take account of the mountainous killer seas of that ocean at that time of the year. There is a brutal monotony in the bitter, shrieking winds, and momentous grey rollers which stretch to the horizon. If high enough on the bridge it is possible to see rollers approaching from several miles ahead, and if one's bows are into the wind each grey sea comes roaring over the forecastle as the ship plunges her sharp end into yet another grey-green wall of cold Atlantic misery. If broadside on to the seas, the sickening rolling has to be experienced to be believed, a monotonous agony of repetitive movement. Working on deck is made miserable by the stinging spume blown off the rollers, to a background cacophony of wind screaming through the rigging. To this day, I feel glad I am on dry land.

Sometimes we sailed in an eleven- or twelve-knot convoy, when some of the ships could only make seven knots all out, and sometimes less. The stragglers had then to be left, and we watched them disappear slowly astern, often encountering them still plugging away at three knots as we passed them on our return journey with a new convoy. It was a time of dreary monotony and prolonged strain, let alone the ever-present menace of the underwater enemy waiting to pick off the juicy, big, careless strays. When one of these happened to be an ammunition ship, the destruction was terrible to see. Time and time again we approached the New World closely enough to clearly hear the United States short-wave radio broadcasts, the music and chat and Americanisms sounding so exciting – yet so far away. Then we would pick up another convoy and come back home again, leaving it all behind once more.

Finally we did enter Halifax, and it seemed Heaven – all those lights, all that food and all those goodies. We stocked up on tinned food, chocolates, nylon and silk stockings, sugar and whatever else we could lay our hands on.

I have said that the *Rodney* was in need of a refit when the War started – the refit was postponed, of course, but the ship was troubled by recurring concerns for water-tightness. Early in 1940 the ship's forward side began 'panting', which caused a certain amount of leakage. The effect was greatest in the watertight compartments below the lower deck, between the two foremost watertight bulkheads. The ship's artificers welded one beam from frame to frame athwartships in this region but the compartment continued to leak due to defective riveting. The trouble was aggravated later by the effect of two near misses when the ship suffered prolonged air attacks during the Norwegian campaign of April 1940.

The seizure of Denmark and Norway was a classic Hitlerian gamble in which he once again successfully staked his own ruthlessness against the irresolution of his enemies. The advantages of Norwegian bases for German commerce raiding are obvious – for example the fjords provided shelter for both the *Bismarck* and the *Tirpitz* at different stages of the conflict. As the war hotted up with the coming of spring, Admiral Forbes's five heavy ships (*Rodney* (Flag), *Valiant*, *Warspite*, *Renown* and *Repulse*) were almost immediately involved in the first moves of the Norwegian campaign, the British ships being thrown into battle at a brisker pace of activity than ever before.

The sea fighting off Norway was confused, the early encounters showing the superiority and greater elan of the Royal Navy over its German opponents. Once the initial invasion impetus was spent the German commanders showed a remarkable lethargy in the conduct of individual actions. The German 'Operation *Weserubung*' called for the participation of almost every active warship available to convey troops and support those landed. In Norway the groups were allocated to Narvik, Trondheim, Bergen, Kristiansand, Arendal, Oslo and Egersund; and in Denmark to Kurso-Nyberg, Copenhagen, Middelfart, Esbjerg and Tyboron. Lack of landing craft required disembarkation at proper harbours, hence complete surprise was essential. The various naval actions included the destroyer *Glowworm*, which rammed the *Hipper* before sinking, the *Renown* which brought the *Gneisenau* and the *Scharnhorst* to an abortive and reluctant action and the Norwegian coastal batteries which sank the heavy cruiser *Blücher* with much loss of life. The *Lützow*, coming to her assistance, was badly mauled. The *Lützow* was further damaged by a British submarine which also blew her stern off. On 13 April Admiral Whitworth directed the *Warspite*'s 15" guns, as she proceeded up the fjord blasting away, and the devastating effect is now part of history. British destroyers also joined in the mayhem. Whenever a German destroyer appeared through the haze and gunsmoke it was obliterated by another salvo. Other enemy destroyers were scuttled by the Germans, who do seem to love scuttling their own ships. Every German destroyer was wiped out. Admiral Whitworth later wrote: 'The cumulative effect of the roar of the *Warspite*'s 15" guns reverberating around the mountains of the fjord, the splashes and bursts of the great shells, the sight of German ships sinking and burning around them, must have been terrifying.'

Earlier, the Home Fleet was experiencing its first taste of determined and prolonged bombing by Luftwaffe units, comprising 47 HE 111s and 41 Ju 88s. The German bombers located the British ships at about noon on 9 April, some sixty miles off Bergen, in clear weather and with no fighter protection. For many hours these ships were obliged to bear the brunt of this prolonged attack. The attacks began at noon and continued until late evening. Years later I saw a newsreel film of the *Rodney*, which again and again turned away so that the German bombs fell just where she *had* been. Considering that the *Rodney* took some time to answer to the helm, the ship-handling of Captain Dalrymple-Hamilton that day was masterly, and we were not hit by any of the high-level bombs. There were only near misses. The only British warship sunk by this prolonged onslaught was the destroyer *Ghurka*, although the cruisers *Southampton* and *Glasgow* were damaged. AA fire was ineffective. Those damned 4.7s made the most unholy noise – a beastly, earsplitting 'crack' – but other than that didn't achieve much. Fortunately most of the bombing was high-level – the least effective form of air attack on ships – unless they are stationary. As was the *Tirpitz* on 12 November 1944, when sunk at anchor in a Tromso fjord, by Wing Commander Tait's Lancasters.

During an engagement, those working below decks – engine room, ammunition supply, transmitting stations, etc. – have little immediate knowledge of what is going on above them. The muffled bangs, roars, jolts and shakings are meaningless unless the men are kept informed. The only unmistakable noise is the characteristic bangitty-bang, bangitty-bang of the multiple pom-poms (Chicago pianos), a distinctive rhythm of eight bangs in two sets of four, this being an indication that enemy aircraft are coming in close, as torpedo bombers or dive-bombers. The good Captain, with his mind on very many things of urgent and pressing importance, tries also to keep those below decks informed of the state of the action. Down in the 4.7 high-angle ammunition magazine, the only direct communications we had, or needed really, was the exhortation to 'Keep them coming' which informed us we were still in the thick of it, of course. Otherwise, we could only eavesdrop on the messages and comments from the ADO (Air Defence Officer) to other stations.

For the group of men beavering away at opening ammunition boxes, sending shells up in the hoists and shifting empty boxes out of the way, there was just one long iron ladder up to the hatch providing exit from the magazine. I did my best to stay as close to the foot of the ladder as I could, but so did everybody else! At the slightest danger that that flash or fire might reach the magazines – 16", 6" or 4.7" – the magazine would have been flooded. There is no chance of escape; the magazines and shell-rooms' crews are drowned like rats in the onrush of sea water as the stopcocks are opened. Yet we may have been ordered to 'Abandon Ship' and I wanted to be close to that flaming ladder!

There seemed no end to the insatiable demands of the high-angle gunners and we were beginning to run out of room for manoeuvre in the confined space. Empty boxes had begun to pile up and it needed considerable agility to dodge around them while carrying a heavy shell. The incessant demand 'Keep them coming' went on and on. Towards evening there was a lull, after having been closed up at 'Action Stations' for some six hours or so. The ship's company began to relax and below decks we had time to make a better disposition of the empty boxes. Then there came the distinctive pre-speech hum of the communication speakers fitted to the deck head, and then the short message from the ADO, 'Single aircraft starboard bow' – there was an urgency in his voice. The plane approached over the bows of the ship, an anti-aircraft blind spot. The pilot released his bomb with great accuracy, it being variously described as 'like a bloody pillar box' and 'resembling an Austin Seven'.

The well-aimed bomb just missed the octopoidal (the eight-sided tower bridge structure). The ADO in the Air Defence Position, atop the octopoidal, yelled out a warning and went flat on his face. Someone on the bridge yelled down to the high-angle guns' crews alongside the funnel, 'Clear the gundeck!' Everybody dived for cover as the bomb whistled down and banged on the edge of a ready-use ammunition locker. These are stout iron boxes, with a small supply of shells, as their name implies. It transpired that the glancing impact cracked open the casing of the bomb, which carried on to pierce the upper deck and the main deck. It broke up on passing through the 4" armour of the latter deck where it partially detonated as a slow explosion, a short, sharp conflagration without the confines of an intact casing. Minor damage was inflicted on surrounding structures by bomb splinters and blast and a fire was started in the galley flat (a 'flat' is a deck level). The port forward 6" gun turret was put out of action temporarily and there were eighteen minor casualties. On the bridge, the Commander noticed black smoke pouring out of the hole in the high-angle gun deck and informed the ship's company, 'We appear to have been hit by a small incendiary,' since there had been no explosion, the ship was still proceeding and the guns were still firing. 'Some incendiary' coughed the men choked by the fumes and singed by the spread of flame. Other less delicate comments abounded. A later BBC announcement that 'A heavy bomb has bounced off the armoured deck of HMS *Rodney*' also came in for some profanity.

There remained the problem of removing the unexploded portion of the broken bomb. It was secured to a stout line and carefully lifted out of the compartment through the hole by which it entered. The captain of a destroyer in company saw the bomb coming down and said it looked 'gi-normous'. Nearly four years later, he joined the *Rodney* himself. An unconscious midshipman, who had also been burned, had his life saved by an able seaman groping around in the smoke-filled space. He felt something soft, with a cupboard lying across it. Heaving the cupboard off the body he dragged it outside into clearer air, in which it began to recover, eventually recovering completely. Mac (he of the Madeira ukelele) was the trainer of one of the port side 4.7 high-angle guns, and at the command to clear the gun deck leaped off his platform but caught his ring finger in a projection – which didn't give an inch. With his finger fixed to the gun he could only wrench his hand away, so that the ring stripped flesh from his finger before breaking, partially exposing the tendons beneath. So much for the *Rodney*'s famous 'bouncing bomb'.

Operations at ground level did not go well. Poorly equipped troops were landed without proper plans, and were soon retreating in the face of German troops and armour, supported throughout by dive-bombers, in turn covered by fighters. Eventually only Narvik remained in Allied hands, and by early June events further south – the collapse of Belgium, Holland and France, and evacuation of the BEF at Dunkirk – led to the abandonment of Narvik, too. The Navy had provided the Army with the only support it had, taking heavy casualties while doing so. Several British warships assisted in the evacuation of our troops as the abortive and confused campaign more or less died on its feet. The *Rodney* had covered many of the convoys landing troops and it was sad to have to help in the evacuation. The Navy had also put ashore a small landing party whose task it was to cover a crossroads, with a machine-gun and ample ammunition. When orders were received to abandon the post and get down to the landing stage for evacuation, they refused, exclaiming, 'Not on your Nellie! Leave all this for the Jerries? Not bloody likely!' and stayed where they were. Nobody knows what happened to them.

Some of the soldiers ('brown jobs') we evacuated were attached to the Green Howards who had to leave much material behind as the enemy advanced in strength to their positions. Almost all of the 'brown jobs' who came off on the *Rodney* were wearing excellent quality sheepskin coats (soldiers, Arctic, for the use of). These luxurious garments were coveted by the guns' crews in exposed positions –

accordingly, military stores ended up on naval backs, and many of the gunners began capering about the exposed gun positions in these quite magnificent sheepskin coats.

Here I might mention the occasion when the lower deck was cleared so that all hands could be addressed by the beloved Captain Dalrymple-Hamilton. We were carpeted, in fact. Life was real and life was earnest, and it was very difficult to keep smart. It had become the thing to make what is known these days as a 'fashion statement', and some of the get-ups were a bit far out, to say the least; fancy sweaters knitted by wives and girlfriends, motley scarves and weird, assorted headgear. The Captain stood on a promontory of the bridge and spoke of his displeasure at the rapidly deteriorating 'scarecrow' appearance of the men, which could no longer go unremarked. 'For heaven's sake smarten yourselves up,' he roared. 'You look like walking jumble sales, like a mob of tramps. I do not enjoy commanding a crowd of scruffy Waterloo station pigeons!' Thereafter the standard improved a bit – for a bit. But one needed something more than the regulation kit to keep out the monotonous cold and the wet.

Following the collapse of the Western Front and evacuation of the British Expeditionary Force from Dunkirk, the prime consideration was the imminence of the expected German invasion of Britain, no fanciful idea since tugs and barges were being assembled on the continent's Channel coast. Together with many other naval units in the summer months of 1940, the *Rodney* was kept standing by, at Rosyth. In some ways this was a disappointment, as we would have liked to came further south. Shore leave was given but everybody had to be back on board at 6.30 p.m., and it was only the possibility of imminent action that made this waiting time bearable. Various exercises were initiated to keep us sharp, among which was a body of Royal Marines masquerading as enemy parachutists, and also the formation of a company of seamen to strengthen the shore defences – should Rosyth be included in the enemy's plan of invasion. The seamen's company was kept in a constant state of readiness, and had to stand by during *all* air raids, of course. Their equipment had also to be instantly to hand, and many of the ship's passages were festooned with this equipment. The Commander of this force, Captain Teek of the Royal Marines, boasted that he could have got his men ashore, fully equipped, within fifteen minutes, and they could have remained self-sufficient for forty-eight hours.

The months of July, August and September passed with *Rodney* standing by for the invasion – the likelihood of which began to fade as autumn, colder weather and rough Channel seas precluded such an undertaking. While the heavy units of the Fleet waited in tense passivity for the most part, young men on both sides of the conflict were dying in the skies over southern Britain and the Channel. The Battle of Britain was a truly revolutionary conflict, in that for the first time since powered flight, aircraft were the instrument of a campaign designed to break the enemy's will and capacity to resist, without the support or intervention of armies or navies. Hitler's 'Directive' to the *Luftwaffe* chiefs, on preparation for a landing operation against England, was stark: 'Prevent all air attacks, engage approaching naval vessels, destroy coastal defences, break the initial resistance of land forces and annihilate reserves behind the front.' Soon after the initial skirmishes Field Marshal Goering reinforced the aims imposed by Hitler: 'The Führer has ordered me to crush

Britain with my Luftwaffe. I plan to have this enemy on his knees, so that occupation of the island can take place without risk to our troops.'

The risks of the air offensive began to loom larger than anticipated, but:

a) The *Luftwaffe*'s operational basis had to be hastily improvised as they were redeployed to the coastal areas of France and Belgium. The RAF operated from well-established home bases.

b) RAF pilots bailed out over friendly territory. Enemy pilots bailed out onto enemy territory or into the Channel.

c) The short-range enemy planes had to fly some 20-100 miles before engagement. RAF fighters could engage as soon as they reached operational height.

d) Fighter Command, operating close to its own bases, enjoyed a highly prepared and integrated early warning system of radar.

e) Fighter Command enjoyed one more advantage – a higher output of fighters from the aircraft factories.

The Luftwaffe might have achieved air superiority had it operated to a coherent plan, but it had no considered strategy and fought the battle by a series of improvisations. The Battle of Britain reached its climax during mid-September days of blue skies and bright sunshine, with hundreds of raiders making for London and being intercepted by British fighters rising to meet them and break up the massed formations. On 15 September some 250 Spitfires and Hurricanes intercepted the German squadrons well east of London and by the end of the day had shot down nearly sixty of them. It was the

Luftwaffe's heaviest defeat – the rest is history. The pragmatism of 'Stuffy Dowding', the skill and self-sacrifice of his fighter pilots and the advantages of radar had inflicted on Nazi Germany its first defeat.

With Germany's abandonment of invasion plans, the Navy could turn its attention and resources to the unremitting Battle of the Atlantic. The important statistics are easily stated. In 1939, the United Kingdom needed to import 55 million tons of goods by sea to sustain its existence. It maintained the largest merchant shipping fleet in the world, of 4,000 ocean-going vessels and large coastal vessels. By way of protection for this fleet the Royal Navy deployed over 200 vessels equipped with 'ASDIC' (Allied Submarine Detection Investigation Committee) echo-sounding equipment, which was not always as effective as believed.

Although attacks by German aircraft and surface ships did sink a certain amount of Allied shipping, the real battle at sea was between convoy escorts and U-boats. Casualties were heavy; 75 per cent of U-boat crews fell victim during the War. Nevertheless, the prospect of enemy surface raiders – *Admiral Scheer, Gneisenau, Graf Spee, Scharnhorst,* and later the *Bismarck* and the *Tirpitz* – roaming the sea routes and preying on Allied shipping was a constant preoccupation of the Admiralty. There is little that a merchant ship, even armed with 6" guns, can do to avoid destruction by a professionally crewed warship which mounts 11"-15" gun turrets, and after wrecking one convoy can escape at high speed to get amongst another spread of slow merchant ships and wreak the same one-sided destruction.

The presence of British cruisers in the South Atlantic – the *Cumberland* in the Falkland Islands, and the *Achilles* (NZ

105

ship), *Ajax* and *Exeter* some 150 miles off Montevideo, together with other dispositions such as ships patrolling the Faroes passage and the Denmark strait – made manifest the dire need to hunt down and eliminate these surface commerce raiders. For the same reason, the *Rodney* accompanied North Atlantic convoys for some months after the threat of invasion had receded. With the approach of winter 1940, these trips became not only monotonous but uncomfortable. The weather varied from bitter squalls off Iceland and, when spray froze as it came inboard, to calmer seas and weak sunshine; but for the most part the 'Winter North Atlantic' weather was decidedly hostile.

During December 1940, some of the gales were a bit too much for the *Rodney*; the old lady was getting on in years. The ship encountered a particularly heavy gale, which she rode out head to wind at about 7.5 knots. While the rolling motion was unexceptional, the pitching motion was pronounced. Each time the bows crashed down into the succession of heavy rollers, it was with a bone-jarring thump, like 'hitting a milestone'. The repetitive force eventually wrenched away the crossbeam previously fitted by the ship's staff. Leakage increased to the extent that two watertight compartments were flooded. During the heavy weather the covers of the navel pipes, by which anchor cables are led below, were ripped off by the sea and water began to enter the cable lockers, which were flooding faster than the pumps could remedy it; two of the pumps were out of action anyway. By further complications, water entered the torpedo tube compartments and then into the drain tanks in the hold. A further leak developed on the starboard side at platform-deck level, just below the muzzles of 'A' turret's guns. This water could only be pumped out by a hose carried through a normally shut watertight door and then down through a hatch in the platform deck – both apertures being a risk to the watertightness of the ship. We went into dockyard hands yet again, on 18 December at Rosyth, where the damage was rectified and the ship's structure stiffened.

We were soon back on the North Atlantic convoy beat, and during March 1941 the *Rodney* came close to catching one of the surface raiders – the *Gneisenau*, under command of Vice Admiral Gunther Lutjens – and bringing her to action, but it was not to be, at least not then. *Rodney* was covering two large convoys off Newfoundland, sailing in company of the more westerly of the two groups of shipping. Reports began coming in of surface raider attacks some 250 miles to the south-east. This more easterly of the two convoys was in the greater danger, although too far away to be reached in time to prevent sinkings.

Vice Admiral Lutjens in *Gneisenau*, in company with *Scharnhorst*, had made use of his two supply ships – *Ukerman* and *Ermland* – to comprise a quartet of ships each separated by thirty miles, thus covering a swathe of ocean 120 miles wide in search for convoys. The advance elements of convoy HX-114 were encountered some 200 miles to the south of Cape Race in Newfoundland. The *Gneisenau* immediately made prizes of three tankers and sank one other vessel by gunfire. The *Scharnhorst* sank two other vessels. Another, slower section of the convoy was following on behind, and the coming of daylight revealed that the German pocket battleships were literally in the middle of the convoy – which promptly scattered. But for nine of the ships it was too late and they were sunk.

The *Demeterton* sent distress signals and other ships followed. The signals received by *Rodney* on 16 March indicated that the enemy was sinking independently-routed eastward-bound merchant ships. One of these, the 1,800-ton MV *Chilean Reefer*, the smallest of the group, was intercepted by the *Gneisenau*, which opened fire on her as she was tapping out the 'RRR' signal. The little ship stood her ground and began to make a fight of it, with her circa 1914 ex-Japanese 4" pop-gun. This was some thirty-three miles to the south-east of *Rodney*. It took an astonishing seventy-three of the German pocket battleship's full-calibre shells to send the brave little US ship to the bottom, the range eventually closing to around 1,000 yards.

The signals ceased and she was not heard from again. The *Rodney* steamed for her last reported position and shortly afterwards a merchant ship was sighted, this turning out to be a German auxiliary. Soon after that another was seen to be on fire, and then a third vessel alongside, momentarily discernible against the evening sky as a warship. The *Rodney* itself was probably silhouetted like a mountain against the fading light from the west. After a brief 'What ship?' was signalled to the warship, and an ambiguous reply received, we began chasing both auxiliary and warship, which immediately picked up their heels and rapidly disappeared into the gathering darkness. As ever, the pocket battleship was happy to sink merchantmen, but not, for the most part, to come to action with other warships. Not having the speed to catch either of the enemy ships, the *Rodney* returned to the burning, sinking wreck and picked up twenty-seven men from an open boat. About thirty minutes before, the boat had been alongside the *Gneisenau*, which left in too much of a hurry to assist them on board. The *Rodney*'s 16" guns posed a threat to Lutjens that he was not prepared to challenge, and he had a narrow escape. Some two months later, on 27 May, Lutjens did meet his fate at the hands of the *Rodney* and *King George V*, while in command of a surface raiding fleet comprising the *Bismarck*, *Prinz Eugen* and associated supply ships involved in Operation *Rheinubung*. Lutjens was killed on the *Bismarck*'s bridge in vain pursuit of Grand Admiral Raeder's belief that the pocket battleship could destroy Britain's sea trade more effectively than the U-boat.

Yet the surface raiders *had* clocked up a resounding success. In just two days the *Scharnhorst* had sunk six ships of 35,080 tons and the *Gneisenau* seven of 26,693 tons. Also, three tankers, adding a further 20,139 tons, had been taken as prizes. The suicidal Allied policy of convoy dispersion had again made these easy pickings for the enemy. The later, disastrous Russian convoy PQ17 well makes the point.

Despite the repairs in Rosyth during December 1940, leaks developed again during March 1941, with a new leak appearing in the hold below the torpedo-body room. The ship's side was still panting and the propulsion machinery was beginning to give trouble. The boilers needed an overhaul and the condensers required new tubes. Nevertheless, the demands of convoy escort required the *Rodney* to continue providing 'heavy unit' cover, so we carried on pounding the North Atlantic beat. The routine became monotonously familiar. We would depart from the Clyde, or Scapa Flow, with a destroyer screen, which after some days out left us to proceed alone, having been shepherded through the greatest concentration, or likely concentration, of U-boats. We would then rendezvous with the convoy we were to cover and wallow slowly across the Atlantic for Halifax. Sometimes we turned round short of the New World – not even sighting it – to pick up an eastbound convoy and start the wallowing all over again. Sometimes we went into Halifax, a welcome break with its lights, food, shopping and girls.

The Battle of the Atlantic continued unabated, but fortune smiled on the Allies to give us a most helpful new shot in the locker. On 9 May 1941, Captain Baker-Cresswell was commanding the destroyer *Bulldog*, leading the 3rd Escort Group, which was shepherding convoy OB318. The German U-boat *U110*, commanded by notable U-boat ace Kapitan Leutnant Fritz-Julius Lemp, who sank the liner *Athenia* on the first evening of the War, had just sunk two of the convoy's ships when its periscope was sighted by the corvette *Aubretia*, which dropped a pattern of ten depth charges. The destroyers *Bulldog* and *Broadway* also got firm Asdic contacts and were just about to attack when sudden violent water turbulence and eerily large bubbles appeared between the two escort vessels. The U-boat broke surface with men pouring out of the conning-tower. Baker-Cresswell prepared to ram and then changed his mind, ordering his own guns to be manned as the U-boat's crew began firing on his ship. For a minute or so there was bedlam, then the firing ceased and *Bulldog* began picking up survivors, which did not include Julius Lemp. Some accounts describe him swimming back to the stricken U-boat and trying to clamber back on board to prevent *Bulldog*'s crew getting into the submarine – he was promptly shot. The survivors were quickly herded below decks, assuming that their U-boat had been sunk. They saw, and were told, nothing. Convoy OB318 steamed onward and out of sight, as a party from *Bulldog* boarded and methodically stripped it of all they could remove – binoculars, sextants, books, logs, charts, diaries, pictures, tools and instruments. A telegraphist noted down all the tuning positions of the radios in the wireless office. The *Bulldog*'s whaler had to make several trips back and forth, loaded with treasures. To Baker-Cresswell's bitter disappointment, the U-boat suddenly sank next morning in the worsening weather; the attempt to tow her back to UK thus failed. But the cryptanalytical gains provided by the stripping operation were beyond price. They included the *U110*'s Enigma cypher machine with settings for 9 May still on its rotors, the special code settings for 'high security (*Offizierte*) officers only' traffic and the current code book for U-boats' short-signal (*Kurzsignale*) sighting reports. Baker-Cresswell was awarded the DSO for capturing this major and profoundly significant prize, by which German signal traffic could now be read. Experts from Bletchley Park, the cryptanalytical centre, went up to Scapa Flow to meet the *Bulldog* and when they saw the two large packing cases of highly secret code-breaking information they could hardly believe their good fortune. The *U-110* yielded information which was to have a major influence, not only on the war at sea but on the North African campaign, too.

It is of interest that Baker-Cresswell was previously the *Rodney*'s navigating officer for three happy years, and was twice commended by their Lordships for his skill in piloting that famously unwieldly ship in and out of harbour.

The story of *U110*'s capture was kept secret for many years, eventually being published in 1959 by the official naval historian, Captain Stephen Roskill. When investing Baker-Cresswell with his DSO, King George VI said that *U110*'s capture was perhaps the most important single event in the whole of the war at sea. Throughout the war the *Kriegsmarine* refused to believe that Enigma had been penetrated. The official revelation, thirty years later, numbed the critical faculties of many interested parties. Admiral Karl Doenitz, the *Kriegsmarine*'s U-boat Chief and eventually Germany's leader on Hitler's death, was shattered when the penetration of Enigma was officially confirmed to him before he died in 1981.

Baker-Cresswell died in 1997.

It was soon evident that a major refit for the *Rodney* could be delayed no longer. Accordingly, in mid-May 1941, she sailed for the USA and the Boston Navy Yard, shepherding a single large troopship westward across the Atlantic. By reason of having to break off and join in the hunt for the German battleship *Bismarck*, we didn't make Boston until June.

CHAPTER VI

The Bismarck *Action*

Since Germany is part of continental Europe, with its ample road, rail and river/canal transport systems providing the means for rapid exchange of goods and people across national boundaries, it is not virtually dependent upon merchant shipping to supply its needs, as is Britain. Moreover, the extent of its coastline is very much less than the extent of its land borders with neighbouring countries – France, Belgium, Holland, Luxembourg, Denmark, Poland, Austria, Switzerland and Czechoslovakia. Hence the necessity to repel hypothetical invasion by sea, and to ensure vital seaborne supplies, is not imperative for Germany as it is for the island kingdom of Great Britain.

The *Kriegmarine*'s emphasis, manifest in its shipbuilding programme, on submarine warfare and surface commerce raiding, clearly indicates that the primary impulse for its maritime force remained commerce raiding and not offensive or defensive surface action against other navies. Thus the construction of two massive battleships – fast, well armed and well armoured, and conceived before the War – were more a matter of national pride and prestige than a vital necessity for Germany's very existence. Nevertheless, these two ships – *Bismarck* and *Tirpitz* – had the potential to perform some pretty effective commerce raiding, and this naturally engaged the Admiralty's interest in them. The cost of the two ships, neither of which it transpired ever did sink a merchant ship, could have bought three 'pocket' battleships, no doubt. It was the potential of these two ships which gave the Admiralty so much concern.

In Volume III of his history off *The Second World War*, Winston Churchill remarked: 'Had she escaped, the moral effect of her continuing existence, as much as the material damage she might have inflicted on our shipping, would have been calamitous. Many misgivings would have arisen regarding our capacity to control the oceans, and these would have been trumpeted around the world to our great detriment and discomfort.'

On 18 May 1941 the Admiralty was informed that *Bismarck* and *Prinz Eugen* (a cruiser) had left Gdynia in the

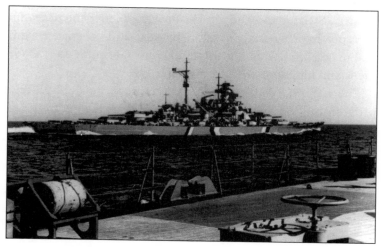

17. Bismarck under way (Imperial War Museum).

Baltic with a heavy escort of destroyers, minesweepers and aircraft and had passed via the Skagerrak into the North Sea. On receipt of this excellent piece of intelligence from the British Naval attaché in Stockholm, the Admiralty made a determined effort to locate and then keep in touch, by sea and air, with this powerful new force. On 21 May Coastal Command found the two ships in a fjord on the south-west Norwegian coast. The fact that the *Luftwaffe* was reconnoitring in northern waters between Norway and Greenland with unusual intensity, and had been doing so for ten days, prompted the Commander of the Home Fleet, Admiral Tovey, to prepare for a breakout of major German units and to make rapid dispositions for British naval forces to prevent these vessels from escaping into the Atlantic. Coupled with the unusual frequency of high flying over Scapa Flow, there seemed no doubt of German intentions. The 8" gun County Class cruiser *Suffolk* was despatched to patrol the Denmark Strait between Iceland and Greenland, to be followed next day by her sister ship, the *Norfolk*. The First World War battlecruiser *Hood*, the modern battleship *Prince of Wales* and six destroyers were despatched from Scapa Flow to Hval Fjord, near Reykjavik in Iceland, while the Town Class cruisers *Birmingham* and *Manchester* were sent to patrol the gap between Iceland and the Faroe Islands.

Admiral Tovey remained at full readiness in Scapa Flow aboard his flagship *King George V* with five cruisers and five destroyers which were also at full readiness. A military convoy in the North Atlantic, destined for the Middle East, was divested of its escort – the battlecruiser *Repulse* and the aircraft carrier *Victorious* – which were placed under Tovey's command.

Bad flying weather grounded the Luftwaffe on 22 May but did not prevent Commander Rotherham of the Fleet Air Arm completing a perilous low-level reconnaissance over the Bergen coastal area, confirming that the German ships had sailed. The German Operation *Rheinubung* had begun when *Bismarck* and *Prinz Eugen* sailed from Korsfiord, near Bergen, Norway for the Atlantic.

If these ships could have joined the *Scharnhorst* and *Gneisenau* at Brest, the *Kriegsmarine* would have possessed a powerful fleet in the Atlantic, which could have wreaked havoc among any merchant fleet group it encountered, and could have given a good account it itself had it been intercepted by British heavy units. It also had the speed to avoid confrontation should it have wished to do so. Compared to the three old British battlecruisers capable of catching them, these German vessels were modern. No wonder the Admiralty considered it imperative to intercept and destroy *Bismarck* and *Prinz Eugen*.

On 22 May the *Rodney*, with four destroyers and the liner *Brittanic* sailed from the Clyde for Halifax and her ultimate destination, Boston in the USA. She was to be taken in hand for a much needed and long-delayed refit.

Since the latest Luftwaffe reconnaissance reports had found the Home Fleet, or some of its units, still at Scapa Flow, Vice Admiral Lutjens decided not to 'waste time' on completing refuelling but to make a quick break out and take advantage of the fog banks reported north of Iceland. During the day and night of 23 May *Bismarck* and *Prinz Eugen* raced at 24 knots skirting westward along the edge of the ice between Greenland and Iceland.

The thick overcast weather concealed the two ships at first

but on the evening of the 23rd the *Suffolk*'s radar, not needing to rely on vision, picked up a contact. Then two German ships loomed out of the mist, seven miles away. A 'MOST IMMEDIATE' signal was sent off and the hunt was on. *Bismarck* opened fire on the *Norfolk*, forcing her to turn away under a smokescreen, and then tried to shake off her pursuers by a strategy of course changes and hide and seek through the fog banks. The two cruisers tenaciously hung on just beyond the range of *Bismarck*'s guns.

Cryptanalysts aboard the German battleship were able to decipher *Norfolk*'s reports and other British signal traffic, giving Lutjens a good picture of the Admiralty plans to cover attempts at eluding the British forces. Further Admiralty measures included instructing Force 'H' at Gibraltar – a battleship, the carrier *Ark Royal* and a cruiser – to move out into the Atlantic and cover an important convoy. Also, the battleships *Ramilles* and *Revenge* were ordered to leave their Halifax convoys and steam east at best speed.

We on the *Rodney* were almost two days out when news was received that the two German ships had been sighted in the Denmark Strait. We were recalled with three of the destroyers to provide additional cover should the German units elude the major ships of the Home Fleet. The *Brittanic* was left to continue accompanied by the destroyer *Eskimo*. *Rodney* was agog with the possibility of real action at last. There was also trepidation, since *Bismarck* was a formidable package and would not be a pushover if it came to confrontation. Some 300 miles to the south, patrolling the south-west coast of Iceland, was the *Hood* (Vice Admiral's Flag), *Prince of Wales* and four destroyers – originally there were six but two had been detached to refuel in Iceland. At

19.54 hours this force increased speed to 27 knots and steered 295 degrees on an interception course. At 03.40 hours on 24 May course was altered to 240 degrees to converge with the enemy; speed was increased thirteen minutes later to 28 knots. 'Action Stations' was ordered at 05.10 and at 05.37 the *Prince of Wales* signalled 'Enemy in sight at seventeen miles'.

It is necessary to briefly consider the fitness of the *Hood* for action against a modern battleship. Known for decades as 'The Mighty *Hood*' she had been the pride of the British Fleet for over twenty years. Conceived in 1914, her design was radically altered after the heavy British losses at Jutland in 1916. She was launched in August 1918, yet some twenty-two years later was as untried in battle as her adversary. She could do a knot or two over the *Bismarck*'s speed, had an unladen displacement of 48,000 tons and was as good to look at as the *Bismarck*. Yet her armour did not bear comparison with that of her adversary, as with all British battlecruisers, and it was totally inadequate for a capital ship with heavy guns as her main armament. Her main weaknesses were her age and her design. As Van der Vat had aptly put it, 'She was an almost perfect microcosm of the British Empire – ancient, glorious, the biggest in the world, shrouded in ceremony and veneration – but out of date and full of defects ... this gleaming grey symbol missed modernisation between the wars because she was in constant use to fly the flag in distant places, maintaining the gigantic bluff which was the latter-day Empire and the myth of her own invincibility.' She was also, in passing, a rotten seaboat and her quarterdeck was often completely awash in anything like a moderately heavy sea.

When the *Rodney*'s Captain announced over our

loudspeakers that the *Hood* and *Prince of Wales* had intercepted the *Bismarck*, there was great excitement and anticipation. We expected not to be required to lend a hand since the 'Mighty *Hood*' was on the scene and would soon 'sort the *Bismarck* out', we confidently expected. Not much was known of the *Prince of Wales* but at least she was fast, modern and powerful. We were not aware that she had not been fully worked up yet, nor had she got over her initial teething troubles. Civilian engineers of the manufacturer were still on board making adjustments to the machinery, having not had time to get ashore before she hurriedly departed for the Denmark Strait. The fact that the *Hood* was on the scene made things a foregone conclusion, of course. Plainly, the *Bismarck* was 'in the bag'.

In the Denmark Strait, action was imminent. With the *Prince of Wales* on her starboard side, the *Hood* approached the enemy at such an angle that only her forward turrets could be brought to bear. There was a defect in one of these guns, which was only able to fire in the first salvo, yet it was important to get as close to *Bismarck* as possible, as soon as possible, so that the effect of plunging fire on poorly protected decks could be minimized. At 05.49 both ships turned 20 degrees to starboard, slightly increasing the angle of approach. Vice Admiral Holland ordered fire to he concentrated on the left-hand ship, wrongly identified as the *Bismarck*. It was the *Prinz Eugen* of course.

The *Prince of Wales* gunnery officer realized this and shifted target to the right. This mistake was realized in the *Hood* a few seconds before opening fire, at 05.52 hours, followed thirty seconds later by the *Prince of Wales*. *Bismarck* opened fire on the *Hood* at 05.55; the first salvo was short, the second over and the third was a straddle. *Prinz Eugen* had also begun firing.

Prinz Eugen scored a hit which started a fire among the *Hood*'s ready-use ammunition on the shelter deck. At 06.00 hours when the range was down to 14,500 yards, Holland ordered his ships to turn 20 degrees to port, so as to bring their full broadside to bear. At this point, *Bismarck*'s fifth salvo straddled the *Hood*. A sheet of flame roared skywards from the base of the mainmast, followed by a tremendous explosion which broke the ship in two. The stem half sank quickly while the fore part took some three minutes to go under. There were three survivors from the complement of 1,418 officers and men. One of them, Briggs (1985), described the moments on the *Hood* before the action.

> The ship began to shudder as speed was raised to 28.5 knots, the maximum she could obtain from her engines after months of overuse. From the billows of blackish-purple smoke emitted from the stacks, there was no doubt that 'the Chief Stoker was sitting on the safely valves'. She was at her fastest and not another decimal of a knot could be coaxed from her ageing engines ... this was no false errand ... doubts that a full-scale naval action was about to be fought were dispelled at once. We would soon be upon the enemy ... there was no friendly conversation on the bridge ... everyone was staring at the steely blend of sky and sea towards the northern horizon ... from the control tower the gunnery officer bellowed 'Shoot' and the warning gong replied before the *Hood*'s first salvo belched out in an ear splitting roar, leaving behind a cloud of brown cordite smoke ... within the next two minutes the *Hood*'s foremost turrets managed to ram in six salvoes each at the *Bismarck* ... suddenly it intrigued me to see four star-like golden flashes, with red centres, spangle along the side of the

Bismarck ... those first pretty pyrotechnics were four 15"
shells coming our way ... the express train increased in
crescendo and passed over-head ... the two German ships
rapidly became more visible and continued winking at us
threateningly ... not far from our starboard beam there were
four high splashes of foam, tinted with a dirty brown fringe.
Then I was flung off my feet. My ears were ringing as though
I'd been in the striking chamber of Big Ben ... agonised
screams of the wounded and dying emitted from the voice-
pipes ... wild cries of 'Fire' from voices pipes and telephone
... I began to feel a great anger at the enemy.

As the *Hood* turned 20 degrees to port 'X' turret roared its
approval but 'Y' turret remained silent. Then a blinding flash
swept around the outside of the compass platform ... lifted off
my feet and dumped head first on the deck. The ship that had
been a haven for me for two years was suddenly hostile ... she
listed slowly to starboard ... righted herself ... only for me to
be terrorised by her sudden horrifying cant to port ... on and
on she rolled ... reached an angle of 45 degrees ... there was
no need to order abandon ship ... it was not required. The
Hood was finished and no-one needed to be told that.

Briggs was sucked deep below the surface then blown up to it
again in a huge bubble of air 'which shot me to the surface
like a decanted cork in a champagne bottle'. Despite the most
careful subsequent post-mortems (two) which were held
about that action, none of the three survivors could recall
hearing a loud or catastrophic explosion.

One week before the 25th anniversary of the Battle of
Jutland (1916) the *Hood* blew up just as three battlecruisers
had blown up in rapid succession in the earlier action.

Prince of Wales now attracted the concentrated fire of the
main and secondary armament of both German vessels, and

at about 06.02 she took a direct hit on the bridge. After about four 15" hits from the *Bismarck* and three 8" hits from the *Prinz Eugen*, and with an entire quadruple turret paralysed by another mechanical failure, the *Prince of Wales* put up a smokescreen and turned away from the Germans, some 7.5 miles away. This decision was prompted by the fact 'A' turret had jammed and was partially flooded. 'Y' turret was out of action and several of the 14" guns had jammed in elevation. Yet the vessel had stood up well to the pounding and had inflicted what was to become the wound initiating the sequence of events leading to the *Bismarck*'s destruction three days later. One of the *Prince of Wales*'s shells had damaged the *Bismarck*'s fuel tanks, causing contamination by sea water. This was enough to prompt Lutjens to call off the proposed merchant shipping strike and to make south for Brest in France. *Prince of Wales* had straddled *Bismarck* with her sixth salvo and did so several times before breaking off the action. The problems with her main armament were entirely the result of mechanical breakdown, and errors in drill, and not the result of enemy action.

Bismarck continued on her south-westerly course, shadowed at a respectful distance by the *Norfolk*, *Suffolk* and *Prince of Wales*.

With the luxury of hindsight, away from the pressing emotional tensions of naval action, Van der Vat considers Vice Admiral Holland's mistakes. The first was to throw away his superiority in firepower of his two ships by opening fire too soon. His second was to advance in close order, with only a few hundred yards between his two ships, and the third was to wrongly identify *Prinz Eugen* as the *Bismarck*. Lastly, by opening fire at a range of over thirteen miles

Holland exposed the *Hood* to plunging fire, always a danger to inadequately armed ships. After her first salvo *Prince of Wales*, brought into service before a proper chance to shake down, lost one of her six forward guns to mechanical breakdown.

When we were told that the *Hood* had been sunk, with very few survivors, the bottom dropped out of our world – we had gone with a numbing shock from elated anticipation to the most awful gloom. Britannia didn't rule the waves that fateful day. It was a severe blow to morale, and people went about their work in a daze of speechless depression. Next day, Sunday the 25th, we heard that all contact with the *Bismarck* had been lost. The *Rodney*'s Captain decided to alter course to the south and to try and get between the enemy and the French ports, for which she seemed to be making. On Monday the 26th we got the welcome news that the German battleship, without the *Prinz Eugen*, had been located by a Catalina aircraft. The aircraft was almost out of fuel so was relieved by a Swordfish from the *Ark Royal*, which had come up from Gibraltar. Hope began rising again. *King George V* (C-in-C Home Fleet) had now joined the *Rodney*.

Devastated by the fate of the *Hood*, which was to shock the British public as the loss of no other warship, Admiral Tovey was determined to seek immediate revenge. Altogether nineteen major warships from cruisers upwards, together with more than a dozen destroyers, were looking for Lutjens. Practically everything that could float or move was now out to get the *Bismarck*.

The Captain kept us informed – that *Ark Royal*'s aircraft were shadowing the *Bismarck*, about the initial, abortive torpedo attack when our planes attacked the *Belfast* by mistake, the second attack on the evening of 26 May, when 'no hits' was mistakenly reported, the awful feeling that the *Bismarck* had slipped through the net, and then the joyous news that she had actually been crippled and was now unmanoeuvrable. We were going to catch her at last! Then came the news of Captain Vian's torpedo attack with destroyers.

We closed up at 'Action Stations' that night. There was little sleep, little conversation. No one wished to talk of anything but what the dawn would bring The C-in-C in *King George V* had decided against a night action. The *Bismarck* was perforce turning in aimless circles, no longer under control of engines or rudder, since this had been jammed at 12 degrees by the last Swordfish torpedo attack. Yet her main

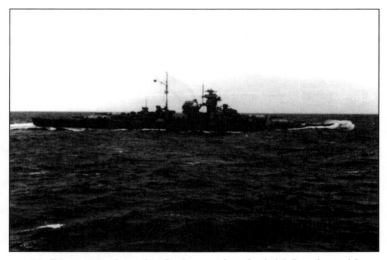

18. Bismarck *down by the bows, after the initial action with* Hood *and* Prince of Wales *(Imperial War Museum).*

armament was intact and the Germans had a reputation for accurate initial range-finding.

Soon after 07.30 hours the Captain spoke just three words to the ship's company: 'Just going in.' There was a strong wind and a fairly heavy sea running, the sky was overcast, but visibility was good.

At 08.47 the *Rodney* opened fire with 'A' and 'B' turrets – the battle was on. One and a half minutes later the *King George V* opened up, and a minute and a half after that the *Bismarck* opened fire on the *Rodney*,

Here follows an account from *King George V*:

> ... There is a sort of cracking roar to port – the *Rodney* has opened fire with her 16" guns ... I have my binoculars on the *Bismarck* ... she fires from two forward turrets – four thin

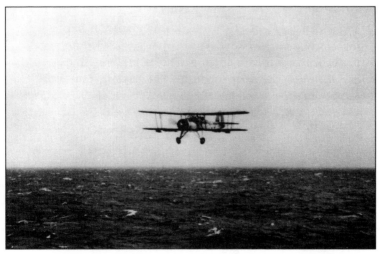

19. A Swordfish from the Ark Royal *returns after successful torpedo attack on the Bismarck (Imperial War Museum).*

125

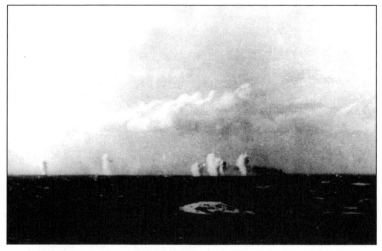

20. Salvoes from HMS Rodney *falling windward of the*
Bismarck *(Imperial War Museum)*.

orange flames. The Germans have a reputation of hitting with
their early salvoes. Now I know what suspended animation
means. It seems to take about two hours for those shots to fall.
The splashes shoot up opposite but beyond the *Rodney*'s
foc'sle. I'm sorry to say we all thought 'Thank God she's firing
at the *Rodney*. . . I watched the *Rodney* to see if she was being
hit but she just sat there like a great slab of rock blocking the
northern horizon and suddenly belched a full salvo. I actually
saw those projectiles flying through the air for some seconds
after they had left the guns, like little diminishing footballs
curving up and into the sky. Now I am sure that four or five
hit. There was only one great splash and a flurry of spray and
splash which might have been a waterline hit. The others had
bored their way through the Krupp armour belt like cheese;
pray God I may never know what they did as they exploded
inside the hull . . . she turned away, then back, writhing it

126

seemed under the most merciless hail of high-explosive armour-piercing shells that any ship, I suppose, has ever faced. There was no escape for the *Bismarck* ... we just went on pumping it out in a steady succession of shattering roars ... the action had been going on for about twenty minutes; some of her secondary armament and two of the great turrets were still firing ... then racing across her quarterdeck were little human figures, running to the guard rails and jumping into the sea one after the other ... we just shot the guns out of her and left her a smoking, lurching, black ruin ... it was like a dog that had been run over.

My own action station was at the base of the octopoidal, the tower bridge structure, and as the shuddering recoil of the *Rodney*'s first salvo rocked the ship, the watertight door from our compartment out to the upper deck bounced off its heavy brass clips and swung open. 'Shut that bloody door'

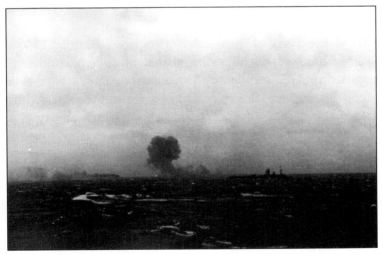

21. Rodney *firing on the* Bismarck *(Imperial War Museum).*

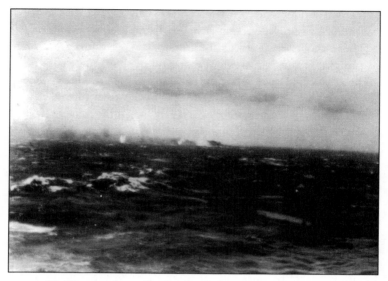

22. Bismarck *on fire in the closing stages of the action (Imperial War Museum).*

roared the Petty Officer in charge of our station. Brown cordite smoke was billowing into the action station as I smartly stepped out (much more smartly than I have ever stepped anywhere, before or since), grabbed the door, swung it closed and secured the clips as firmly as I could. My luck was in – had the *Rodney* fired a salvo while I was exposed on the upper deck the blast would have done for me. There was a stage in the action when the *Bismarck* had almost been silenced and it was safe to gather behind the shelter of the bridge structure and see what was going on. The range had come down to a few thousand yards. The German battleship was an awe-inspiring sight. Her upper deck was terrible to behold – it was a flaming, smoking scrapyard and there was

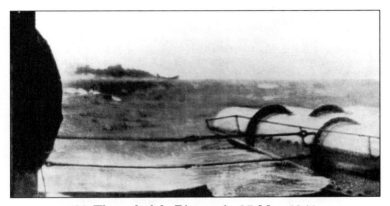

23. The end of the Bismarck. *27 May 1941.*

fire everywhere. She was just full of fire. Fire on the bridge, fire erupting from holes in the upper deck and fire spewing out of holes on the upperworks. Her once menacing 15" guns were drunkenly sprawled every which way. One of her turrets had its back blown out. By 09.02, *Bismarck*'s foretop, the forward fire control station and turrets Anton and Bruno had been disabled – she had lost more than 50 per cent of her firepower. No one in those forward action stations survived.

The senior German survivor of the action wrote a highly detailed and thoroughly researched account of the *Bismarck*'s beginning and her end. He mentions that while in the water, some 150 metres from the ship's side, he surveyed her starboard side from deck to keel as she listed to port, and states that he could see no battle damage. He also mentions floating on the heaving Atlantic like toys, and 'only when we topped the crests of the waves did we catch a glimpse of the horizon'. From his lowly position in the water, he apparently could not see what was plain to observers on the *Rodney*'s

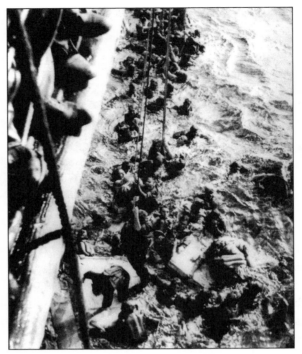

24. Bismarck *survivors being pulled aboard the* Dorsetshire
(Imperial War Museum).

bridge – a great gash on her starboard side, about the level of
the forecastle breakwater, into which the sea poured as she
dipped her bows and out of which it cascaded like a Niagara
as her bows rose out of the water again. It was an estimated
fifteen yards long and about three yards wide. Possibly it was
this break in the forward hull which caused her to be down
by the bows after the initial action in the Denmark Strait.
While easy to sink a merchantman with heavy calibre shells, it
is difficult to send an armoured battleship to the bottom in

this way. British ships continued firing at the *Bismarck*, and we saw one of these shells exploding at the base of the bridge, with a white sheet of flame which shot as high as the top of the structure. There was no redness, no copper glow and no smoke, only this instantaneous sheet of brilliant white flame which must have incinerated, on the instant, everybody on the bridge.

Epilogue

The *Rodney*'s Captain reported ... 'The closing phases of the action were anything but pleasant, but as the enemy had not hauled down his flag there seemed to be no other action open to me but to fire, as it was essential to sink the enemy as rapidly as possible.'

Captain Teek RM, in charge of 'X' turret, at one stage of the action shouted down the voicepipe, 'She's on fire from stem to stern.' The immediate response from those unsighted was, 'Who, sir? Them or us?' – which illustrates how important it is to keep everybody in the picture, especially those below decks.

Raven & Roberts refer to the effect of blast from *Rodney*'s main armament. When 'A' and 'B' turrets were first fired on forward bearings, many weather-deck fittings were damaged and conditions on the mess decks below became very uncomfortable. When 'X' turret was fired abaft the beam, considerable damage was caused to the superstructure and the bridge was untenable, especially when the guns were at high elevation.

An interesting sidelight is afforded by the comments of Marshal of the Royal Air Force, Sir Arthur ('Bomber') Harris who, in 1941, crossed the Atlantic on a mission of aircraft procurement in the USA. He writes:

> I was delighted when I heard I could take my wife and small daughter with me, and still more so when we were offered passage in a battleship, HMS *Rodney* . . . Dalrymple-Hamilton, who commanded the *Rodney* when the *Bismarck* was sunk, gave us an interesting account of the action . . . the *Rodney* closed to such short range that she had in the end depressed her guns so low as to tear up her own deck planking and slightly depressed the steel decking beneath. The *Rodney*'s great guns were still all blistered and peeling and you could see where her deck planking had been patched up . . . apart from this she had no other damage except a hit by one shell fragment . . . it must have been a hair-raising task for this ancient old battle-wagon to wade into the *Bismarck*, especially as this was within hours of the *Bismarck* having disposed of the *Hood* at extreme range . . . The journey took seven days on a zig-zag course, calling at Halifax and arriving at Boston in the dark. I recall the staggering effect, after months of blackout at home, of the lights and neon signs shining miles out to sea.[27]

The effects below decks of successive salvoes was devastating. Ventilation trunks had been dislocated, dust and debris were everywhere, much crockery had been broken and all clothing lockers had burst open and spilt their contents. It was heart-rending to see the damage *Rodney* had done to herself in the living spaces. The force of the recoil of a 16" gun salvo was absorbed not only by gun turret mechanisms but also by the ship as a whole.

The following are extracts from an analysis of the action[9]:

Wind NW, heavy swell, sea rough, sky overcast, visibility good.
First salvo 08.47 fell far right of target.

Two salvoes at 08.48, hits obtained.

Salvo 18 at 08.58(?) hits seen.

Salvo 24 was a straddle.

Hits seen with salvoes 31 or 32.

Salvo 40 seen as a straddle.

Range down to 6000 yards by 09.30 hours – salvoes 61 and 62 were fired.

Hits seen from salvoes 63 and 64.

Hits observed from salvoes 74 and 75.

Hits seen from broadside salvo 94, and subsequent salvoes.

After salvo 98, fire was concentrated along the waterline, and in one consequent broadside as many as five or six hits were observed.

Hits were seen from salvoes 102 to 113, which was the last.

Bismarck was still afloat but extremely low in the water and on fire.

The overall rate of fire during the action was 1.6 salvoes per minute. Shells used were 16" armour-piercing. Exact number of hits unknown but estimated to be forty at least.

With regard to *what* sank the *Bismarck* – shells, torpedoes or scuttling – a letter in the *Daily Telegraph* reads: 'I must state that if she did succeed in scuttling herself it was a quite remarkable feat of timing or chance. As the Observer of a Fleet Air Arm Swordfish crew flying from *Ark Royal*, my pilot and I were circling a few hundred feet above *Bismarck* during her final minutes. We saw *Dorsetshire* approach, fire her last torpedo into *Bismarck*'s port side and within seconds of this hit watched the battleship capsize to port and then founder.'

I fail to understand why the Germans should be so keen on scuttling their ships. In the *Bismarck*'s final situation, what glory is conferred by 'You didn't sink her, we did'? The truth is that the *Bismarck* was a brave ship, which fought under disadvantage to the very end with her colours still flying. Every British ship in the vicinity of her end saluted her and her stalwart men. We just *had* to put her down.

The details were featured in a *Daily Express* report of the action a few days afterwards. According to a German gunnery officer among the survivors 'The *Rodney* knocked seventeen bells out of her.'

The *Bismarck* did little damage to the *Rodney*, and this only from splinters or shrapnel from shells which fell short. One of these chunks of Teutonic ironmongery, about the size of a child's football, came whistling into the octopoidal (the tower bridge structure) penetrating its outer skin and entering the 'meteorological office', a euphemism for the tiny metal cubbyhole in which the synoptic charts were prepared, by me, for the meteorological officer to make his forecasts for our particular patch of the ocean. The shrapnel disintegrated further as it ricocheted around inside the 'office', penetrating several thick books and doing other inconsequential damage. Had I been sitting in my little wooden chair it would have done for me, I think. For years afterwards I kept a two-pound chunk of that German shell, until it became just another piece of shapeless, rusty metal which had long since lost any significance.

About the *Hood*. Admiral of the Fleet Lord Chatfield, living in retirement at Winchester, wrote to *The Times*. . .

The *Hood* was not the most powerful warship afloat. True she was the largest but she was constructed 22 years before the *Bismarck*. In those 22 years engineering science and the power/weight ratio have changed beyond imagination . . . The *Hood* was destroyed because she had to fight a ship 22 years more modern than herself. This was not the fault of the British seamen. It was the direct responsibility of those who opposed the rebuilding of the British Battle Fleet until 1937, two years before the second Great War started. It is fair to her gallant crew that this should be written.

Prinz Eugen, detached by Lutjens after the sinking of the *Hood*, never even began her programme of commerce raiding but headed in a wide sweep out in the Atlantic before turning east for the shelter of Brest.

Being now short of fuel we did not actually see the *Bismarck* sink. By then we were well on the way towards the Clyde and resumption of plans for our refit in the USA. Meanwhile, *Rodney* had most adequately fulfilled the purpose for which she was built.

On return to the UK we signalled to the ammunition depot for a replenishment of 300 armour-piercing shells, only to be politely asked what on earth we had done with our previous stock. News sometimes travelled very slowly.

We returned to the Clyde and stocked up on stores, fuel and ammunition (which had to be removed again before we entered the dry dock at Boston), having tidied up most of the chaos below decks and cleaned up the filth. I was able to get a telephone call through to Barbara in London – it was quite tremendous to talk to her. I didn't know when we would meet again, and it transpired that it would not be until March, 1942, when I left the *Rodney*, after three and a half years on the ship.

Having escorted yet another convoy across the Atlantic to Halifax we had to tie up alongside a wharf, and there were various high jinks trying to get a heaving line ashore, to drag across the heavier line which would secure us to the wharf. The Gunner's Mate had tried twice to shoot the line onto the

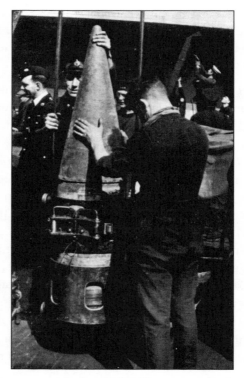

25. Re-ammunitioning with 16" armour-piercing shell.

dockside for it to be grabbed by dockside hands, but the stiff breeze carried it back into the water separating us from the wharf. Taking more deliberate aim with his 'Costain' gun (a gun firing a small rocket to which a line is attached), and gritting his teeth for a more successful shot, the Gunner's Mate got it ashore alright but this time he'd put it through one of the big dock shed windows, thereby raising the sound of much shattering glass and a cheer which must have been heard in Vancouver.

The ship was very quickly infested with newspaper reporters – if some at home had not heard of the *Bismarck* action Canada certainly had.

We left Halifax after a day or two, and made for Boston, going in to the harbour at night. We had not seen such lights for two years or more; they stretched left and right as far as the eye could see. The United States of America, personified by Boston, Massachusetts, was an upturned Horn of Cornucopia of dazzling lights, gargantuan hospitality, food, iced drinks, nylons, girls and wonder – yet I would fain have been in Streatham, London SW16 if truth were told. Having been raised on a diet of American films, in the thirties and forties, we were agog to see what the New World was like. We'd had an introductory taste at Halifax, but not much of a taste. Spread all over the *Boston Globe* newspaper, some days after we arrived, was a feature article on HMS *Rodney* and her sea fight with the *Bismarck* – profusely illustrated. So much for security, yet the presence of hundreds of British sailors in an American port could hardly be camouflaged.

Getting *Rodney* into a dry dock was usually a bit of a squeeze but the one we entered in Boston could no doubt have accommodated the *Titanic* – it was huge! There were the customary wash-houses, latrines and cookhouses alongside the dock (ship's crew, for the use of) but there were two other factors making for an uncomfortable time – the enervating, humid heat of the Atlantic seaboard in the summer months, and the non-stop activity of the American dockyard workers. One began to understand why Americans set so much store by air-conditioning. No doubt the authorities wanted the ship back to duty as soon as possible, but it was at some cost. It was impossible to get away from the rivetting, welding, hammering and general cacophony of dockyard work. Relief was at hand in the shape of a former CCC Camp (Civilian Conservation Corps – part of President Roosevelt's New Deal, dealing with unemployment). The camp was a series of airy, single-storey wooden huts, in a bucolic setting of trees and much other greenery, at Fitchburg, some sixty miles from Boston. Batches of 150 of the ship's company were bussed out there for a week's 'rest'. It was anything but – I recall little of what effect an avalanche of British sailors had on this small American one-horse town but what memories I do have are of sailors and inhabitants getting on like a house on fire. I met a couple of the locals, with two charming daughters of five and six, who couldn't hear enough of the war at sea and the *Rodney* and all about the convoys, between clam bakes, weeny roasts and barbecues, and other hospitality at the Rod and Gun club. Each story got a little more embroidered with each telling, of course. Americans at home are the most hospitable people in the world, and they could not provide enough for us.

One couldn't walk more than a yard from the dockyard gates before a car drew up, a head came out of the window and one was invited to 'Hop in, Limey', and invitations to here, there and everywhere poured into the ship, far more than a ship's company of twice the number could have attended.

In some ways it was doubly sad to hear later that year, in December, the tragic news of the Japanese attack on Pearl Harbour, when war came to those delightful Americans with a vengeance.

For the first, and probably the last, time in our lives we were treated like heroes. The *Bismarck* action was still front-page news and everybody wanted to know everything about it, every detail, as though we had sunk the German battleship all by our little selves. Boston was a delight. There was much turn-of-the-century architecture and earlier period graceful building, and evidence of a rich colonial history in older parts of the town. The transport system was pragmatic – one could go from any part of the town to any other part for the flat rate of ten cents, the tickets being interchangeable on buses, subways and trams as required. What simple sense! Not far away was the famous Harvard University, at Cambridge, Massachusetts. The oldest in America, it was founded in 1636, although not initially as a university. The whole region was rich in colonial history, even unto the Boston Tea Party of 1773.

The New England countryside in summer was very beautiful, but we didn't stay into September/October and so missed those lovely autumnal fall colours. Boston had other charms – the bar at the Copley Plaza Hotel slowly revolved like a roundabout, and there were some (sensible) irritations for smokers, this not being permitted in cinemas, another example of the town's pragmatic arrangements for its citizens' comfort. Our primary memories of Boston were of the hugely warm and natural hospitality of Americans – many would drive hundreds of miles or more to the dockyard, to pick up invitees for a country weekend, or a party, or a dance, a clam bake, weeny roast or beach games.

During late August it came time to leave. We had all been through a wonderful experience, that of a fabulous introduction to America and Americans, on their own home ground. Our departure was marked by a farewell dance given by the ship's company and a cocktail party, attended by some

400 official and private guests, given at the State Hotel by the officers. During the evening the Wardroom was presented with a piano by the Honourable Artillery Company of Boston – to the end of the *Rodney*'s days (1948) that piano stood in the Wardroom. Our ammunition was hoisted back on board again, a 48-hour day-and-night job by 100-foot high cranes.

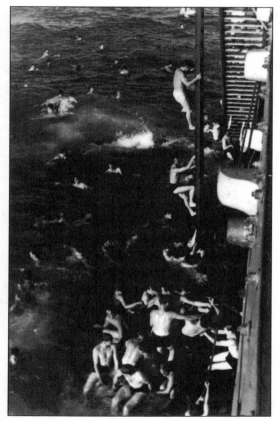

26. Swimming over the Rodney's *side in Bermuda.*

Their accuracy was uncanny. The cordite and shells were picked up from the dockside, slung skywards over the ship and then set down precisely on their allotted space on deck (Fig. 25). As we moved out of the dock and proceeded out of harbour, every single vantage point was crammed with sightseers, for whom this was the first chance of laying eyes on the ship. And no doubt the odd broken or yearning heart among them. The waving continued until we could see them no more. Our first stop was Newport, Rhode Island; then on to Bermuda, where we anchored for ten days in Tobacco Bay. We needed that respite to tidy up below and above decks, to recover from the huge hospitality of those lovely Americans and to have a swim over the ship's side (Fig. 26).

CHAPTER VII

Gibraltar, Malta and Iceland

The ship's company were fortunate to have enjoyed a wonderful six weeks respite from the War, while people at home coped with rationing, the blackout, the bombing and all the dreariness and inconveniences.

We rejoined the War forthwith by way of sailing from Bermuda to Gibraltar, there to become a battleship member of the famous Force H, which had built for itself a terrific reputation as a formidable fighting force. Having carried out an audacious and very successful bombardment of Genoa in February 1941, helped to account for the *Bismarck* (Fig. 27) and covered many battling convoys to the beleaguered island of Malta, Force H had got a name for itself and we felt we were joining distinguished company.

As we approached Gibraltar after sunset it was a perfect blaze of lights; there was no real blackout in comparison to Britain. The place was stuffed to the brim with 'brown jobs' (soldiers) and could put up the most stupendous anti-aircraft barrage. Having known Gibraltar for some sixty years, starting in 1935, it seems to me that the one thing it is good at is being an anomaly! It sticks up from the bottom end of Spain like a sore thumb, is British but not really, the native Gibraltarians are not quite Spanish and there is a frontier

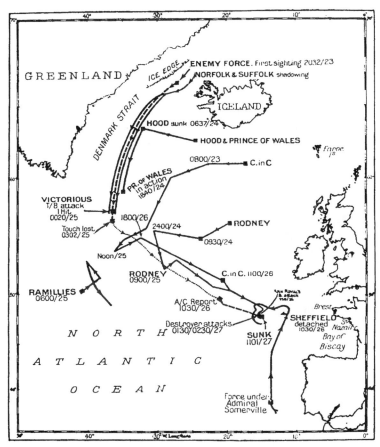

27. *Chart of ships' dispositions during the* Bismarck *action.*

post between 'The Rock' and Spain proper. Brother Geoff and I were fortunate enough to meet up in Gib; I'm not sure now what ship he was on. We met again at Plymouth in 1947, just before he left the RN and took himself back to Rhodesia; I never saw him again.

We could still enjoy the pleasures of doing a little shopping for wives and girlfriends, and avail ourselves of the robust hospitality of the various sergeants' messes ashore. But the War was only just around the comer and we were soon to get a taste of those hectic Malta convoys.

Malta was annexed by Britain in 1814 and subsequently became an important naval base, situated on the route to British India and the Far East. A glance at the map shows the strategic importance of Malta – as an Allied base for operations (air, surface and submarine) against the supply traffic for the Axis Powers and their North African campaign. It was in the interests of Italy and Germany to render Malta inoperative by bombing and to starve it of supplies by preventing Allied convoys from reaching it with food, ammunition, petrol, oil and war materials. The island was awarded the George Cross for its endurance under heavy air attacks between 1940-2, until in October of that year when the British Eighth Army (the 'Desert Rats') began the sustained push which was to drive Rommel's Army either into the sea or into prisoner-of-war camps. During those two years from 1940 the supply line to Malta had to be kept open, and the convoys entailed some bitter fighting and parlous losses on both sides.

All the naval comings and goings at Gibraltar were plain to Axis agents in Algeciras, a ferry port and resort on the Bay of Algeciras opposite Gibraltar. As soon as an assembly of merchant ships and escort vessels departed eastwards through the Straits of Gibraltar, the fact was made known to Rome and Berlin without delay. The vital cargoes to Malta were given every protection possible. Aircraft-carrier protection was provided by the *Ark Royal*, that doughty ship whose Fairey Fulmar fighters tore into the enemy bomber concentrations with such courage. They would give us protection, by the fighters but also by anti-submarine patrols, as far as the Narrows, that war-torn stretch of water between Sicily and Pantelaria; the latter is a small volcanic Italian island between Sicily and the coast of Tunisia. A selected force of cruisers and destroyers escorted the convoy through to Malta. The function of the heavy units ('the heavy mob') i.e. *Rodney*, *Nelson* and *Prince of Wales*, was to take on the Italian Fleet, should it get over its shyness and show itself, and to add to the anti-aircraft barrage that the scale of attacks demanded. The Italian force of battleships was numerically strong enough to overcome easily the British 'heavy mob' but did not attempt to put their preponderance of firepower to the test. Alter several of the earlier convoys, when all of the escort vessels were fully prepared, for all of the time, for whatever might be thrown at them, a certain pattern became evident and a strategy for husbanding resources for the 'busy' times could be worked out. After the initial encounters, when the high jinks began almost while still in sight of Gibraltar, the pattern became: The first day, D-Day, was quiet. On D+1 air attacks began in the afternoon and continued during dusk and sometimes into the night, too. On D+2, air raids were virtually continuous, up to the point when we left the convoy and turned back for home at sunset. During D+3 there would be more air attacks in the forenoon.

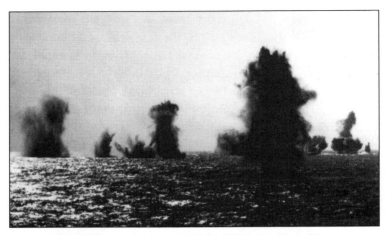

28. Malta convoy early 1942. High-level bombing.

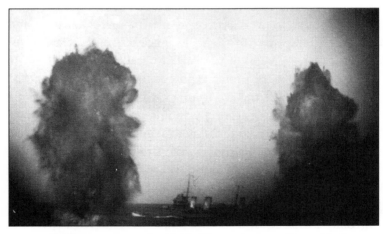

29. Malta convoy early 1942. Near misses on Emerald-class cruiser.

This time the attacks developed as expected, with the first onslaught at about 1400 hrs on D+1. A group of Junkers 88s began bombing the convoy but were soon split up and disorganized by the Fulmar fighters from the *Ark Royal*. A few 88s got through but were met by an AA barrage which effectively put them off. Even the merchant ships were having a go, banging away with their little guns at whatever they believed was in range and could be hit. This was comparatively early in the War and the Fleet Air Arm had not yet received those 'killer' American aircraft, the Grumman Martlet and the Vought Corsair, yet the Fulmars did invaluable work. On D+2 the activity hotted up, mostly from the large Italian S-M three-engined torpedo bombers. This type of attack requires cold courage of a particularly elevated kind. So far as the British Swordfish aircraft is concerned, the pilot must fly straight and steadily, some 90 feet above the sea surface at 90 knots, until 900 yards from the target, when the torpedo can be released. During that time the torpedo bomber had to face not only a 'fire-spitting mountain' like the *Bismarck*, for example, but, later in the War, the main 15" or 16" armament of a battleship used as a 'splash barrage', laid down by the guns firing at extreme range.

Many of the S-M planes were shot down, because they were a large target, yet the Italian pilots attacked with great courage. They were falling into the drink like ninepins. One got through to the *Nelson* and the torpedo struck home, forward on the port side, at platform deck level. A hole some thirty feet long and fifteen feet deep was blown in the outer bottom, causing extensive flooding. The torpedo room was wrecked and the platform deck flooded for a length of seventy-five feet. Speed was restricted to 15 knots to avoid added strain on the damaged structures. *Nelson* remained in convoy for a short period and then proceeded to Gibraltar for temporary repairs. The Italian Fleet was reported to be out and we were detached to chase after it together with other heavy units and destroyers. Being made aware of our intentions the Italians retired to Naples. We rejoined the convoy and the mayhem of further attacks.

There was a world of difference between the Malta convoys and those of the North Atlantic in winter, or the Russian convoys, when every danger was compounded by the bitter, lethal cold. The Mediterranean was invariably calm and the visibility good with blue sky and sunshine. The various forms of Axis attack were high-level bombing, dive-bombing, torpedo-bombing, submarine attacks and E-boat attacks, the latter in the Narrows, of course.

Later convoys were more hectic. After I had left the *Rodney*, the convoy of August 1942 (Operation Pedestal) – which I experienced by way of a Gaumont British Newsreel in the comfort of the Odeon cinema in Streatham, London SW16 – was the mother and father of a battle. Not for nothing was the Mediterranean known as 'Bomb Alley'. *Rodney* and *Nelson* were again engaged in this, the greatest Malta convoy of them all.

By reason of lack of oil supplies, the six Italian battleships remained in harbour, and the task of destroying Operation Pedestal was left to the Axis air forces, strong submarine patrols and numerous E-boats stationed in the Narrows. The escort vessels comprised *Rodney* and *Nelson*, the fleet carriers *Victorious*, *Indomitable* and *Eagle*, the old carrier *Furious* to fly off fighter aircraft for Malta, seven light cruisers and thirty-one destroyers, as well as corvettes, oilers and a fleet tug, to

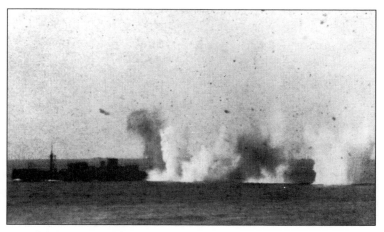

30. Malta convoy August 1942. Some near misses on a tanker in company with HMS Rodney.

escort the convoy of fourteen merchant ships. Against them were ranged 320 Italian and 227 German aircraft, 18 Italian and 3 German submarines, 19 Italian and 4 German E-boats, plus a cruiser squadron. It was a hard, bitter battle.

The convoy passed through the Straits of Gibraltar on 11 August and the first air attacks took place later that day. The German submarine *U-73* put four torpedoes into the *Eagle*, which was left sinking. Battle recommenced early the next day and the convoy forged doggedly ahead, beating off numerous bomber and submarine attacks. Destroyers sank two U-boats and many aircraft were shot down. One destroyer had been damaged and the *Victorious* slightly damaged but the *Indomitable* had been badly bombed. The greatly outnumbered Fleet Air Arm fighters could not stop all of the bombers from getting through but the enemy planes which did then had to face the greatest AA barrage ever

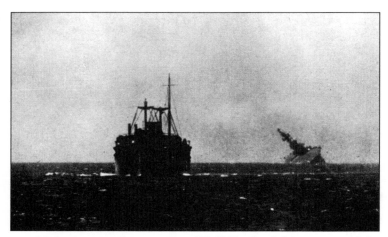

31. Malta convoy August 1942. HMS Eagle *sinking astern of the* Rodney *after sustaining four torpedo hits.*

mounted by a British force to date. The 16" gun 'splash barrage' laid down by the *Rodney* and the *Nelson* deterred many of the torpedo bombers from coming in any closer, but one such aircraft kept pressing on through the splash barrage, the destroyer screen barrage and the small-arms close-range flak. It was badly hit, with all engines on fire, before the torpedo was released.

A minute later it hit the sea in a cloud of spray and debris. A Junkers 87 (Stuka) dropped a large bomb some twenty yards from the *Rodney*'s port side – happily it failed to explode. Simultaneous torpedo-bomber attacks, dive-bombing and high-level bombing kept the guns' crews fully occupied while the destroyers and corvettes kept the submarines from getting too close. As Smith (1977) described it: 'And on throughout that blazing hot summer's day, with the clear blue Mediterranean sky pock-marked with flak bursts and scarred by trails of flaming aircraft, the bright sunlit sea burst asunder by bomb, torpedo and depth charges.'

Rodney's log of bombs, aircraft shot down, torpedo attacks and other assaults, on 12 August, makes interesting reading. Just regarding torpedoes alone, it illustrates the savagery of the action:

0745 Two torpedoes pass ahead. We comb their tracks
0953 Track of torpedo crosses bow from port to starboard
1015 Torpedo passed ahead from starboard
1045 Torpedo passed astern from port bow
1245 Torpedo dropped on port bow
1246 Six torpedo bombers on port beam. Appeared a number of torpedoes dropped.

The log continues to record close action during the afternoon and evening. Not included are the numerous other entries of high-level and dive-bombing during the morning and continuing throughout the day. At dusk on the 12th, when the heavy units turned back, the convoy had lost no merchant ships. During the night the E-boats struck and sank several ships, escorts as well as merchantmen. By day the bombers were active again but no Italian warships bigger than an E-boat appeared. Five of the merchant ships got through to Malta, their cargoes keeping the island going till the end of the year, by which time the Mediterranean scenario had changed dramatically.

After the last convoy (Operation Halberd of September 1941) when I was still serving on the *Rodney*, we did one more quick run to Malta with the *Furious*, which flew off Spitfires, and then left Gibraltar for England, with some survivors from the destroyer *Cossack* and some prisoners of war from an Italian U-boat. It was all very well to have had an intriguing one-off break in Boston, USA for six weeks, but it was not the same as leave to go home and see loved ones. We had not had any leave for ten months and were longing for a trip home and a real break. But we had to wait for a few more months yet.

After disembarking our *Cossack* survivors and Italian submariners we set out to sea again from Scapa Flow, this time for Iceland. There, in Hval fjord at Reykjavik, we formed part of the heavy unit force waiting for the *Tirpitz*, sister ship of the *Bismarck*, to venture out from her anchorage in a southern Norwegian fjord.

My recollections of the time between our departure from Gibraltar and my leaving the *Rodney* at Liverpool in March 1942, are hazy. Some events and emotions of that period are clear as a bell, others are vague. One little cameo, as crispy-clear in my memory as the day I observed it, happened during one of our trips between Scapa Flow and Iceland – I don't recall whether we were coming or going. We accompanied an aircraft carrier (whose name has long since sunk without trace) which was flying off regular anti-submarine patrols by Swordfish aircraft. It was a very windy day with a turbulent sea, and as the relief patrol had just taken off we watched the previous patrol landing on, with the usual destroyer in close attendance. Just as one aircraft had been signalled by the 'batman' to cut its throttle and land, the stern of the carrier yawed abruptly away to one side, leaving the Swordfish suspended in mid-air without flying speed. It plummeted into the ship's wake like a brick, and floated for a few minutes. The destroyer came tearing across to the carrier's wake like a greyhound out of the starting trap, and in no time had plucked the pilot and observer from the bitterly cold sea. I had never before seen such instant response – it was quite heart-warming.

During the winter of 1941-2, Winston Churchill had sent a memo to the Chiefs of Staff Committee: 'The presence of *Tirpitz* at Trondheim has now been known for three days. The destruction or crippling of this ship . . . (would be) . . . the greatest event at sea at the present time.' There must have been other considerations governing strategy of the Allies, since the presence of *Tirpitz* at Trondheim was not known until about 22 January 1942. Most of what the *Tirpitz* achieved was by her mere existence, because she pinned down Allied forces – mostly British – whose combined strength greatly exceeded her own. The German strategy was thus sound and it was to be almost three years before Wing Commander Tait's Lancasters and Barnes Wallis's 'tall-boy' bomb finally put paid to the German battleship, which was left capsized in Tromso fjord. She had crept south after an earlier raid had severely damaged her bow. Like her sister ship, this expensive warship never did sink even one merchantman. Meanwhile, dispositions of Allied forces were made to cover the possibility of her attempting a *Bismarck*-like breakout into the Atlantic and the vital shipping lanes.

With us in Hval fjord was the US battleship *New Mexico*, together with other units of the American Navy. One noteworthy incident in an otherwise very boring and dreary sojourn, was the visit to the *Rodney* of Douglas Fairbanks Jnr., then serving as a Lieutenant Junior Grade on what he called 'a middle-aged American destroyer'. Later during that time in Iceland he served as a lieutenant on the *USS*

Mississippi a battleship and the flagship of US Task Force 99. Looking very dashing in his naval uniform, he toured the *Rodney's* mess decks, addressed the ship's company over the sound reproduction system, cracked a few good jokes and generally did a very good public relations job.

Towards the end of November 1941, the *Mississippi* was ordered home to the US Naval Base at Norfolk, Virginia, and Fairbanks gives a graphic description of winter at sea in the North Atlantic, with mountainous seas and force 9-10 winds, inflicting much damage to upper-deck structures and much water-sodden misery below decks, for two or three days. Several members of the American ship's company were incapacitated by injuries received during the storm's battering of the battleship.

Iceland was not a lot of fun, either for the natives of the small town of Reykjavik or the servicemen based ashore as well as on the Allied warships in the fjord. The time spent in Iceland was just about the worst of the whole war, for the ship's company. There was little to do ashore, even if we could get there, since Hval fjord was a little distance from Reykjavik. It was virtually an Allied occupation of the country, when the servicemen of two nations suddenly swamped the bewildered, peaceful Icelanders. The small, neutral civilian population, the very short winter days so far north, the dreary cold and the dull scenery, the great lack of recreational and social facilities and the absence of any kind of foreseeable end to the period of our incarceration there – all added to the potential explosive force of a powder keg. On inspecting the shore through binoculars, one of Fairbanks's colleagues remarked, 'Well, I can understand why we are here in Iceland, and I can understand why the British are here in

Iceland, but I'll be goddamned if I can understand why the Icelanders are in Iceland.' This ancient and highly schooled civilization produced some of the most comely people in Scandinavia, of whom the women were particularly statuesque. But opportunities for fraternization with the local young ladies was much restricted, and the local people were understandably resentful of a situation which obliged them to put up with thousands of Allied soldiers, sailors and airmen. It wasn't that they preferred the Germans, they just wanted to get on with their lives without falling over alien personnel at every step. Difficulties and tensions were compounded by the really good-looking Icelandic women, who were remarkably pretty and occasioned many a fight for their attentions. And thereby hangs a tale.

The local population were shocked and profoundly angered when it was disclosed that two sailors (UK or USA, I do not know) had gone ashore and raped an Icelandic girl. This stupid, mindless trespass was felt as an affront to the whole community, who thereupon imposed complete social ostracism of naval personnel. Official business and purchasing in the shops was continued but with icy formality. When sailors did get ashore (since it was henceforth very restricted) the local people virtually ignored them. It was related to me 'They don't even bother to look away, they just look right through you, as though you're not there.' But one Stores Chief Petty Officer had made a social niche, of a kind, for himself by 'flogging' service issue boots to the Icelandic farm girls, since the volcanic soil was pretty hard on footwear and new supplies difficult for civilians to obtain. His price was not money but sexual favours. Yet, he complained, ostracism continued during copulation. 'They might just as well be reading the share prices in the *Financial Times* over your head while you are performing, for all the interest they take in the proceedings.' But during one encounter, things began to liven up a bit, it seemed. His partner began to writhe around, squirming and making little grunting noises, and wrapping her arms and legs about him with an element of enthusiasm. He was chagrined to discover that all she was doing was trying on the boots. He wasn't getting so far ahead after all.

I must confess to a stupid breach of regulations. As the meteorological assistant it was my job, among others such as taking weather observations etc., to decode tabulated information from the UK on weather reports from shore stations and ships and to plot the information in symbolic form on synoptic charts. These were used by the meteorological officers to draw in the isobars and thus have the information to make forecasts for our sea areas of operations. I had access, of a not very important kind, to maps, charts, forecasts and so on, and made the mistake of keeping a diary, which was quite naturally forbidden. It was entirely for my own information and interest but was still a diary. One day I left it about – someone found it and turned it in. Without my being aware of the investigation, it was traced to me. One afternoon, when I was having a nap on one of the mess-deck benches I was tapped on the shoulder and told to accompany the Master-At-Arms i.e. the Chief 'Crusher' or ship's policeman. With a sinking feeling in my belly I was taken below and put into one of the ship's cells – with a guard outside to see I didn't saw through the bars with my concealed hacksaw, no doubt! This felt like the very end. The dull, boring misery of Iceland, the beastly hostile weather, the lack of daylight, the lack of leave, and now this. Foolish me – I had expected someone to stumble across the diary sooner or later and wasn't all that concerned. I should have been. A very serious view was taken of the matter and for a little while there seemed to be some suspicion that I may have had dishonourable motives, or something of the kind. As I have indicated, the whole atmosphere, on the *Rodney* at least, was something of a powder keg, and consequently my possible motives were very thoroughly scrutinized. Some ten days later, when it had no doubt become obvious that I was a fool rather than a knave, I was released from my cell (in which, incidentally, I had enjoyed my Christmas dinner 1941) and was charged, on the upper deck in front of a section of the ship's company, with keeping a diary. I lost a good conduct badge, was taken off the meteorological duties which I enjoyed and was told, in effect, not to be such a bloody fool in future. And that is the end of the story, except that one wall of the cell was the ship's side, and I was down there during one of our trips between Iceland and Scapa Flow. A U-boat scare induced the usual drill of destroyers tearing about the ocean dropping depth charges. These horrendous bangs sounded and felt as though they were just outside the cell wall. At the first totally unexpected 'boom' the sentry outside the cell shot up the steel ladder like greased lightning. We both thought the ship had been torpedoed, in which case the bowels of the ship were no place to be, if we had no action station down there. I yelled out 'What about *me*?' and he came down again, mumbling 'Sorry, mate, it was just a reflex action.' So after that we commiserated with each other while the bangs continued, he outside the cell and me in it. Someone had yelled down the ladder, 'They are depth charges.' I missed my interesting duties in the Met Office but I had brought it all on myself. We are so often the architects of our own difficulties and tribulations.

In March of 1942, we entered the familiar Gladstone Dock at Liverpool and were at last given leave. Among a group of about 150 of the ship's company, I was drafted to the Naval barracks at Devonport and so left the *Rodney*, after three-and-a-half years on that great lumbering monster.

The train ride from Lime Street station, Liverpool, to London passed as in a dream. I could hardly believe I would soon be seeing my Barbara again. She looked so lovely – I could not believe she had lived in London all through the bombing and the blackout and the rationing and the dreadful endless need for fortitude and endurance. Next day we took a bus to Kew Gardens where I asked her to marry me and she said 'Yes'. We were married on 21 July 1945 at Wandsworth Register Office and as we stood outside for the photograph the sun came out. We had forty-six lovely years together.

★   ★   ★

As I have mentioned, the next time I saw the *Rodney* was in 1942, in an Odeon cinema in Streatham, London SW16. The ship went on to give valiant and valuable service for another two years or so, even though she was virtually worn out by her own exertions and the storms she had weathered. She escorted a convoy to Freetown, Sierra Leone and during that trip crossed the equator for the first time in her history. She was active in a shore bombardment during the North Africa landings and in 1943, together with *Nelson*, *Warspite* and two aircraft carriers, she operated east of Sicily to protect invasion forces. In September 1943 she supported the Salerno landings and bombarded defences at Reggio; and was also much occupied in beating off German torpedo-bomber attacks. She was present at the surrender of the Italian Fleet on 9 September. Back in home waters for D-Day 1944, she bombarded shore defences with *Warspite, Ramilles* and a monitor. Later in June, she bombarded enemy tank concentrations *seventeen miles inland,* to the great discomfort of a German armoured division. The uncanny accuracy of her target pinpointing was achieved with a spotter aircraft, and the armoured vehicle concentrations were very effectively broken up.

As a tail-piece to this – some forty years later, after I had long since left the service and had gone back to school, training as a Chartered physiotherapist, I was in private

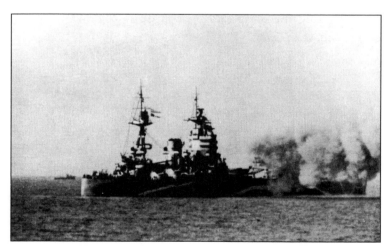

32. Rodney *firing her main armament in support of troops attacking* Caen.

manipulative practice in Halesworth, Suffolk, and to one of my patients I had mentioned, in casual conversation, times past and the *Rodney*. It transpired that he had landed in Normandy on D-Day and later was fighting his way towards Caen. His army group were up against heavy German resistance and prospects looked pretty bleak. He and his companions kept hearing express trains passing overhead and could not think what it might be, until it was revealed that the *Rodney*'s 16" shells were tearing through the air to land among the German concentrations of armour. The old lady also bombarded German gun batteries on the island of Alderney, before going north to escort a Russian convoy to Murmansk. The presence of *Tirpitz* still constituted a threat. In 1944, *Rodney* finally creaked and groaned her way up to Scapa Flow for the last time, there to cease her wanderings and become the static Flagship of the C-in-C Home Fleet. She was sold for scrap and broken up in 1948, as was her sister ship, the *Nelson*.

Historical Note

It had become the fashion to decry the value of battleships in modern warfare, yet they did sterling work, the variety and integrity of which can best be judged by briefly summarizing the war career of one of them – HMS *Rodney*.[16]

September 1939, at Scapa Flow with sister ship *Nelson*, three R-class battleships, battlecruisers *Hood* and *Repulse*. October 1939 heavy air attacks on *Rodney* and others in North Sea. Until end of November occupied on patrol in North Sea, intercepting enemy shipping, searching for German raiders, including the *Gneisenau*, and escorting important iron-ore convoy from Norway. After Scapa was proved unsafe, operated from Clyde and Lock Ewe; suffered mechanical problems, rejoined the Fleet in the New Year, returned to Scapa when base made secure. Struck by heavy bomb during Norwegian operations in April 1940; fifteen casualties. Covered and assisted in evacuation of British forces from Norway. During period of most intense commerce raiding, winter 1940-1, with *Nelson* covered the Icelandic-Faroes passage. January 1941, hunting *Scharnhorst* and *Gneisenau* in North Atlantic and Arctic. Also covered convoys, picking up survivors from those mauled by German battlecruisers. Sighted enemy briefly and gave chase, but *Scharnhorst* and *Gneisenau* slipped into Brest. Covering another convoy when called away for the *Bismarck* hunt. Covered her possible line of retreat into Bay of Biscay, then ordered out when *Prince of Wales* and *Repulse* forced to seek fuel in Iceland. Joined *King George V* and scored her first hit on the *Bismarck* with her third salvo. Given freedom to manoeuvre (unlike *Prince of Wales* earlier), escaped damage from *Bismarck*'s guns, then helped reduce her to a floating wreck. Remarkable speed reported to have been achieved by tiring machinery. Flagship of Force H in September 1941, and on hectic Malta convoy with *Nelson*, *Prince of Wales* and carrier *Ark Royal*. When threat of commerce raiding by *Tirpitz*, *Scheer*, *Gneisenau*, *Scharnhorst* and heavy cruisers renewed, joined Home Fleet again. Another Malta convoy in August 1942; very heavy air attacks, during which her 16" guns were used at maximum elevation at a range of nine miles. First shore bombardment during North Africa landings, and in following year (1943) with *Nelson*, *Warspite*, *Valiant* and two carriers operated east of Sicily to protect invasion forces. September 1943 supported Salerno landings, bombarded defences at Reggio; beat off German torpedo-bomber attacks. Was present at surrender of Italian Fleet, 9 September. Back to home waters for D-Day and with *Warspite, Ramilles* and a monitor bombarded German strong points. Later, in June 1944, to German dismay, bombarded armoured-vehicle concentration *seventeen miles inland*, with aid of spotter aircraft. Also bombarded German batteries on Alderney, before going north to escort Murmansk convoy still threatened by *Tirpitz*. Ended the War as Home Fleet flagship at Scapa Flow. Altogether steamed 156,000 miles on war service at sea.

Battleships e.g. USS *New Jersey* and USS *Missouri* were brought out of mothballs to add their considerable weight to the American attack during the Gulf War. These unique ships are now history, and to my mind their best epitaph is the book *The Great Ships Pass* by Cyril Smith (1977), Kimber, London. We shall not see their like again.

CHAPTER VIII

Physical Training, a Sinking and Sierra Leone

On returning from leave I walked tall – my proposal had been accepted by Barbara and I now had a fiancée – officially!

I was immediately drafted to a holding camp on the outskirts of Plymouth, at St Budeaux, where we lived in Nissen-type huts. It was high summer then and the scents of the countryside around the camp were quite beautiful. Nobody had heard of pollution then, in the way it has become a fact of life today, because there was none to speak of – rivers and the air were clean and the fields were free of chemicals, at least by comparison to the present.

And there were no dark satanic mills in Devon.

I was on guard duty one day, which meant standing around at strategic points of the camp, carrying a rifle and trying to look military. Someone had a wireless playing in one of the huts. I shall never forget that beautiful music – Liszt's *Sonatto del Petrarca* No. 123, the piano solo by Anatole Kitain. I wrote to the BBC for the reference number of the record and still have it, an old '78', fifty-five years later. When I eventually read Laurie Lee's *Cider with Rosie*, his poetic descriptions of high summer evoked memories of that delightful day and that entrancing music.

I had got stuck into the business of promotion and moved successively from Able Seaman to Leading Seaman and then Petty Officer. During those weary Atlantic convoys I had begun tackling the educational requirement for commissioned rank and had successfully taken several subjects.

Harking back to 1934 and my days at HMS *St Vincent*, the boys' training establishment at Gosport, my admiration for the Royal Marine Sergeant PT Instructor encouraged me to try and get accepted for the specialist training at the Royal Naval School of Physical and Recreational Training, at Pin Street, Portsmouth. My legs were not all that athletic and I couldn't run very fast but I was like a porpoise in the water and did eventually contest the Inter-Services Diving Championships and the Devon County High Diving Championships of 1947, so I did have something to offer. In passing, while HMS *Excellent*, the naval gunnery school at Whale Island, Portsmouth was known as 'The all-gate-and-gaiters mob', the PT school at Pitt Street was known as 'The all-swank-and-sweaters mob'. My application was successful and late in 1942 I got a train from Devonport and reported to the Pitt Street premises later that day. HMS *Victory*, the naval barracks at Portsmouth, was a forbidding place then and I was relieved to discover that the PT School had its own accommodation huts on a playing field just across the road from the school. It was a strange time. Portsmouth had been badly plastered by the German bombing and there were great gaps in the city's buildings. Everything was still blacked out every night and there wasn't much in the way of entertainment. The one bright spot was a public house, much favoured by the lucky lads of Pitt Street, nicknamed 'The Dragropes' (I forget its proper name) and it was in this hospitable establishment that the landlord's wife used to appear towards closing time with a large meat dish of baked potatoes, at very modest prices. For a ravenous group of young men bursting with muscles and fitness, this was manna from heaven, and we had a high old time stuffing ourselves with beer and baked potatoes, after a hard day leaping about the gymnasium, the parallel bars, horizontal bars, trapeze over the swimming bath and other muscular capers. There was a pre-arranged system for discouraging non-Pitt Street patrons from hanging about, at least on the evenings when the PT trainees were holding office and getting warmed up for the baked potatoes.

The one advantage of Portsmouth was its proximity to London, that is, compared to Devonport. One day, when I was told Barbara was ill, I got a train from the Harbour Station to Waterloo, then a bus to Streatham, had forty-five minutes with my indisposed fiancée, got a bus back to the station and the train to Portsmouth, all in one evening. It was so worth it. Not like those weekend leaves from Devonport, when one got a bus from St Budeaux to North Road Station and then the London train, which seemed to crawl along for ever, it seemed. The only available train for getting back to the West Country on a Sunday evening was the 9.50 from Paddington, the quite awful 9.50. Barbara used to come as far as Waterloo with me on a 109 bus, we'd make our goodbyes under the railway bridge, at the bus stop, and I'd start walking up the slope to Waterloo Station and the Underground to Paddington, either before she'd got her bus back to Streatham or while she was still waiting for it. Of all those dreadful wartime goodbyes, partings under the railway bridge at Waterloo were the worst. We were engaged to be married but there was no kind of certainty that we might achieve a future – things were so bleak. I have never, before or since, known such profound depression of spirit and hope.

The 9.50 used to crawl along in the blackout, the carriages hot, stuffy and smelly in the summer and uncomfortably cold in wintertime. One was turfed out at North Road station in the small hours of Monday morning, with one's spirits on the floor, to wait in the early darkness for the infrequent bus to St Budeaux. That is why Portsmouth was such an improvement.

We were a motley throng, gathered from the three home ports and all with some tales of war experiences so far. The

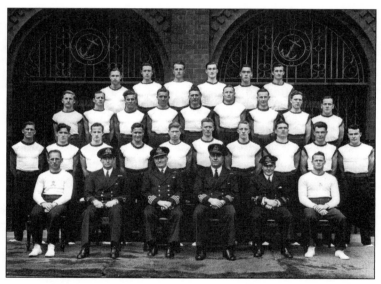

33. RN Physical Training School, Pitt Street, Portsmouth, December 1942. Author standing on right of second row.

group photograph regrettably does not include Colour Sergeant Milton, the dapper little RM PT Instructor who was such a good teacher. He was absent for some reason I cannot recall. There were some original characters among the qualifiers, as we were known, but none more so than Commander Algy Wales, the undisputed boss of the establishment. He was just a natural-born eccentric, who was just as likely to pull up his shirt and show you his operation scar as to take Sunday Divisions by riding on to the gymnasium floor on his bicycle and wobbling unsteadily through the ranks as he 'inspected' the troops. We all loved him dearly, of course.

For those six months, from December 1942 to June 1943, we enjoyed a further respite from the War. We were accommodated as a group, ate and slept as a group, sweated in the gymnasium as a group and suffered aching muscles as a group. We generally made a merry band of brigands who would happily have died for each other. I only ever saw one of them again. Driving along the South Lambeth Road from St Thomas's Hospital in 1963, I came to a traffic junction with a policeman on duty – who should it be but ex-Petty Officer Goodson, also ex-'clubswinger' as the PT Instructors were called. We had a very brief chat as he held the traffic up, until drivers began sitting on their horns and he had to wave me on.

The only piece of apparatus I was quite useless on was the horizontal bar. My trunk is thick and too heavy for my proportionately weak arms, and one needs a good pair of arms to shine on the horizontal bar. Nor was I too good at leaping over box horses. Not enough mobility in the hips, no doubt. Yet each was good at some things and poor at others, or at least indifferent. Towards the end of the course, when the things each of us shone at had become obvious, we put on several circus-like displays at the school – there was no charge but the hat was passed round for charity and we contributed some sizeable amounts of cash to our favourite causes – one of them was a new oven for 'The Dragropes'. Some of the group went down during the War, I know. I nearly did, too, but that comes later.

The course came to an end, and after a final toast at 'The Dragropes' it was time to disperse to our home ports and whatever dispositions awaited us. I hung about for a week or two until I received a draft chit for HMS *Philoctetes*, a harbour base-ship in Freetown, Sierra Leone, of all places. Who would want a Physical Training Instructor in West Africa, for heaven's sake? And on a rusty old bucket, anchored and sweating in the harbour, at that. But there was no argument about it and I was given just 48-hours leave before catching a train for the Clyde and a troopship. I strongly resented devoting several hours of the precious total to crawling along at upwards of two miles an hour on a Great Western Railway train to London. Portsmouth would certainly have been a better bet. I arranged with Barbara that I'd get a Northern Line Underground train as far as Balham and then start walking to Streatham. She began walking towards Balham and we met on Tooting Beck Common. We had a little over a day together before it was time to say goodbye again – Oh! those awful goodbyes. There had been so many of them and each had been like a little death. The interminable rail journey from the barrack platform in Devonport to the dockside at Greenock, on the Clyde, was quite obscene; I was part of a consignment of bodies from the

West Country to West Africa, and our tribulations began on the long, weary train ride, which took the best part of twenty-four hours. Sometimes we crawled along, other times we just stood still for small eternities. By the time we got onto the drifter which took us out to the anchored troopship, we were weary, hungry, dirty, unshaven and not a little angry at this bloody silly war.

Spirits rose when we got onto the troopship, the SS *California*. She was an ex-transatlantic liner of some 17,000 tons, with much of her pre-war supplies still on board and available at the ships' shop. I bought tinned fruit and sugar and things for Barbara, to be delivered sometime, I hoped. The ship also had good, commodious accommodation, which was definitely pre-war in its generosity. She had been converted to an armed merchant cruiser in 1939 and then into a troopship in 1942. After some tidying up, a wash, food and an inspection of our surroundings, life didn't seem quite so bad. It was mid-summer and the banks of the Clyde were very beautiful. The sweet fresh air of Scotland was about and the War receded for a bit. The ship was stuffed to the gunwales with troops – 'brown jobs' – airmen and sailors. We soon shook down and settled ourselves into the accommodation, familiarized ourselves with 'abandon ship' stations and so on, and began to anticipate a sea trip during the next few days, when we might enjoy the air and the vista and spread sideways a bit.

The cargo of bodies must have been considered precious, because we had at least two 'abandon ship' drills before we sailed and another two while under way to Freetown. My own station was to swing one of the lifeboats out and see it lowered into the water. Having completed my duties I would then be free to jump into the boat myself. We were well out in the Atlantic, about opposite Cape St Vincent in southern Portugal, when the 'abandon ship' drill was ordered yet again. This was just getting too much, we thought, but it was no drill. A German Focke Wulf 200 Condor maritime reconnaissance aircraft had spotted us far below, and it began dropping some very well-aimed bombs. We heard our own little pop-guns opening up and then came the shattering 'BOOM' of a heavy bomb, much too close for comfort. That was the one which did for us – we could feel the ship lurch and then begin to tilt. Then came the – this time expected – cry of 'Abandon Ship'. We needed no encouragement – there was an undignified scrambling rush for the upper deck, with me well in the lead. For some reason the ship's siren was giving voice, I don't know why because our predicament was quite plain to the world. The ready-use ammunition of the pop-gun was exploding and sending things whizzing about. There was a degree of pointless running about when the main thing was to get into a boat and get off the bloody ship. I got to my lifeboat and found some disorganization of the boat's ropework – I cannot recall quite what – and it took several minutes to disentangle the mess and get things running freely. With the boat lowered and in the water and pulling away from the ship it was time for me to join it. I took off the 'Burberry' I'd put on when it was plain we'd have to decamp, with a tin of fruit I'd shoved into the pocket. Best thing was to throw it down to the boat first, so I yelled down to my chum, Petty Officer Plum, who was already in the boat, 'Catch my coat, will you.' I clambered down the falls (the ropes by which a boat is lowered), dropped into the drink and swam the few yards to the boat. Soaking wet, of course, I clambered into the boat and looked around for 'Plummy' – who was nowhere to be seen. Then I spotted him lying stretched out on the floorboards, temporarily unconscious and bleeding profusely from a scalp wound – the tinned fruit had hit him on the head! The bleeding looked awful but scalp wounds always do, of course, and he looked much better after a sea-water wipe, which stung a bit, he said.

The boat was pretty crowded because we had a few supernumeraries, and I felt it incumbent upon me to fist hold of an oar and do some pulling away from the ship, which by now was beginning to settle a bit. I hadn't known that the chap on the seat behind me was one of the stokers, who'd received a chest injury from the bomb blast. At each pull, as I leant backwards with the oar, he would groan with pain and it was obvious I couldn't go on rowing like that. So I just sat still and pulled with my arms only. This was very tiring, and soon I couldn't do it any more. In my tired, wet misery I looked up at the darkening sky and saw the star Venus shining over the water like a bright ship's lantern. Will I ever see that star again, I thought? Would the escort vessels find us in the dark, and pick us up? Or would they give it up, as there were U-boats about and the ship was more important than a few men? Would they leave us tossing about on the briny without a friendly ship in sight? I needn't have worried, or more likely should have had more faith. We heard voices – 'Here's another lot' – and how sweet that sounded. One by one we were shifted from the lifeboat into one of the two boats which had found us in the dark. Our rescuers were from the corvette HMS *Douglas*, one of the escort vessels.

Long may she prosper – but probably broken up long since, I expect.

We just found somewhere to curl up and sleep; there were bodies getting long-needed rest in every nook and cranny of the small corvette, as it made its way to Casablanca in Morocco. That experience has given me a much better understanding of what it must have been like to survive a sinking during one of the Russian convoys, when even a few minutes in the water were lethal. A day or two later we entered Casablanca harbour and on looking over the side I saw dozens and dozens of hammerhead sharks, no doubt attracted by the rubbish and waste food thrown overboard. I made a mental note not to fall overboard in Casablanca.

From the time of the first alarm to our being picked up by the corvette's boats, some three hours had elapsed – it seemed more like three years, especially during the time in the boat on a darkening sea. While on the short trip to Casablanca there was another scare – planes, U-boats, surface ships? I cannot recall – but do remember just wanting to be obliterated. I felt I just could not stand any more and nothing was worth going through all *that* again. Yet on many occasions during the War, survivors went through it twice, notably at the German attack on Crete in May 1941, and during a later Russian convoy, when a cruiser which had picked up survivors was itself then sunk, with many of those picked up having suffered twice – in that lethal sub-zero cold. Perhaps I wasn't as durable as I had imagined.

A group of US Army vehicles were waiting at the dockside as we tied up, and having quickly bundled ourselves into these trucks (since we weren't slowed up by possessions – we'd lost them all) we were driven to the US Army camp, a huge place, on the outskirts of Casablanca.

Our reception there was another eye-opener of American

hospitality. We were given a huge meal and then lined up at trestle-tables piled high with underwear, shirts, boots, socks, trousers, blousons, sweaters and small accessories, including toilet gear – we were completely kitted out in US soldiers' uniforms. Our individuality and rank, so far as appearances were concerned, was erased in that excellent quality American clothing. It was a very strange five days. Chief Petty Officers looked just the same as Able Seamen. We were accommodated in large tents, lined up into streets, but not allowed to dwell on our peculiar circumstances or to vegetate. There were organized talks about US policy in North Africa, cinema shows, detailed advice on local infections and diseases and instructions on living under canvas. We were formed into platoons and companies and had to muster two or three times a day to answer roll calls. Given airmail forms on which to write home, we were instructed on what we could write about and what we could not. During instruction there, by an engaging New Yorker whose 'first' always came out as 'foist', I gathered that there were eight US states which began with the letter 'M' and eight beginning with 'N'. He also told us about W.C. Fields's tombstone on which was inscribed: 'All things considered, I'd sooner be here than in Philadelphia'. Those Americans really put themselves out for us. I informed Barbara, in my airmail letter, that I'd had an impromptu salt-water bath – together with the US-style format it should tell her the news, in case there had been some news report which could cause unease.

We all looked forward to being transported home again, for a week or two's leave before the next step, but not a bit of it – we were all transferred to another troopship and sent right on to Freetown. And what a caper that was – our arrival in

Freetown dressed as US troops. We had to announce to the military reception committee who we were and what we were. There were some interesting statements. I just said 'Petty Officer Grieve – Clubswinger' (PT instructor) but others were more exotic: 'I'm Mickey Mouse and I'm looking for Minnie,' 'Greta Garbo in drag', 'King of the United States of America', 'First Lord of the Admiralty', 'Dame Agnes Weston'. My destination was a rusty old bucket of a merchant ship, renamed HMS *Philoctetes*, a base and repair ship for maintenance of the myriad escort vessels using Freetown as a stop for convoys on the way round Africa to the Middle East, Ceylon, India and Burma – not a particularly inspiring posting for a newly qualified and keen young PT Instructor. There were a few old cricket bats in the sports store, some rusty fencing equipment (*everything* eventually rusted in Freetown), an assortment of used footballs and some odds and ends. Not a heartening reception but I got stuck in, polished up the fencing equipment and got some small classes going. Astern of us was moored the *Edinburgh Castle*, another much-used merchant ship which acted as an accommodation unit. It, too, boasted a PT Instructor, Geordie Watson, who was much more interested in football than I was – and was also much fitter than I was. He would break out into voluntary handstands at the drop of a hat, just for the sheer exuberance of living.

There were several sports facilities in Freetown – football and rugby grounds, facilities for tennis, a small dam making a little swimming pool halfway up one of the hills behind the town and two good beaches, among other attractions. Physical and Recreational Officer, Lieutenant (RNVR)

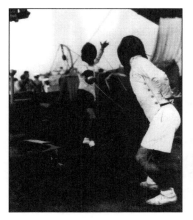 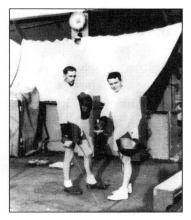

34. Fencing instruction on HMS Philoctetes.

Beswick, arranged a rugger match – Navy versus RAF – which meant HMS *Philoctetes* taking on the denizens of an RAF reach-me-down airstrip some miles away out in the West African bush. He organized a trial game in Freetown in order to pick the Navy side, including me as the full back of one of the teams. He was a front row forward for the opposing side and I have a clear memory of this large muscular forward bearing down on me, the last bastion, with aggressive intent. I stoutly dived to stop him but was swept aside almost as an afterthought, while his majestic progress continued. In later years, I used to boast 'I had a trial for the Navy v RAF once,' but didn't add that the 'Navy' was a rusty old bucket sweltering in Freetown harbour and the 'RAF' was a moth-eaten little airstrip in the West African bush.

The whole affair was, of course, just an excuse for a good old booze-up that evening at the RAF camp where the 'game' was played. The very hospitable RAF chaps put us up for the night. Good thing. We weren't capable of getting back to Freetown after that bash. It was, in fact, a humdinger of a 'sod's opera' and I learnt a few of the RAF's ditties.

Lumley beach was the usual bathing place but there was also 'No. 2' beach which, for servicemen, could only be reached by organizing transport – usually a military lorry of the 'covered wagon' type, open at the rear end. During the trip of several miles over dusty roads, the occupants were soon covered in a fine red dust, stirred up by the passage of the vehicle. One *needed* a dip in the sea on arrival. Going back to the ship entailed arriving on board in dire need of a shower. It was a superb beach and on one occasion a chum and I fixed up the transport and went out to No. 2 beach in a tropical downpour. There was a certain enjoyment in swimming in the sea while being thoroughly rinsed in rainwater. One found oneself doing slightly strange things in Freetown. Swimming in the little dam halfway up the hill was a refreshing change but a difficult climb in the steamy heat.

The prime difficulty in West Africa is the climate – hot, humid, enervating and generating a marked reluctance for energetic occupations. It was fatally easy for the weak-minded to begin to become a little 'coasty' i.e. to become lax about personal hygiene, to get lazy, to take to native women and to get into the state which resembled the desert madness, the *cafard*, of the French Foreign Legion. It was understandable that Sierra Leone is dubbed 'The White Man's Grave'. Across the harbour from Freetown one could see the low-lying Bullom shore, from which a typical weather system, with an invariable sequence, used to emanate. There would be a sudden increase in wind strength, the sky would go heavy and dark and Bullom shore would disappear in a rain squall, which moved rapidly across the harbour towards Freetown, suddenly hitting – literally hitting – the *Philoctetes* with real force. The heavy clouds literally opened up, with a massive amount of water making loud drumming noises on every horizontal surface. It would be impossible to hear speech or shouting, so loud was the cacophony of falling water. The surface of the harbour would boil and a prodigious volume of water would suddenly be deposited on the steaming earth. Just as suddenly it would cease, leaving a sodden, streaming universe to recover its equanimity.

Strange how little pockets of pre-war civilization and plenitude lingered on into the mid-forties. There was a strange little shop in the Barbican, Plymouth, which used to stock fine old crockery well into the war years, when it was virtually unobtainable elsewhere. There were a number of small Asian shops in Freetown and a couple of more ambitious emporiums, which still, in 1944, stocked some of the finest silks and other materials. It was like entering Aladdin's cave to see all this finery after the experience of clothes rationing at home. I bought a whole lot of things: silk for underwear, terry towelling, napkins, tablecloths and other napery, tea towels, bath towels and whatever else was going, happily stocking up for Barbara's bottom drawer. Whenever one of my companions completed his West African stint and was going back to the UK, I would ask him to take a small parcel and post it when he got home, to Streatham, London SW16. A few parcels never made it, but most did, and Barbara's wedding trousseau was of silk from Freetown, as was the terry towelling I am still using today. Typically, I had overbought.

Since one of my duties was to handle outgoing and

incoming mail, I was ashore every day for about an hour or so, by special boat, and so got to know a number of the town's 'officers', as it were. One of these was the chap in charge of the local Cable and Wireless Office, a charming man with an equally hospitable wife and a ten-year-old daughter. Since the daughter liked being read to, and I enjoyed reading, I used to 'baby-sit' for the couple, reading stories to the daughter while they went out for the evening. The arrangement also included a well-cooked meal in civilized surroundings – a great relief from the ship – and served by their native servant. The little girl was something of a dreamer, and as soon as the story started she was lost in her own imagination and her eyes would take on a wide, glazed look. I hit on the idea of getting her to read stories to me, about which she got very enthusiastic; it even began to get difficult to find suitable new stories. I never did know who watched the shop, i.e. who was available to receive messages and cables while the pair were out, but it seemed to be taken care of. There were very few electronic gizmos in those far-off days of half-a-century ago. It was a little touch of home, and I enjoyed those evenings.

While it was vital to keep the convoy system going, and to provide base, repair and hospital facilities for the never-ending stream of escort vessels, it was difficult to avoid the feeling that when great things were happening in the war theatres, we just sweated and got hotter and damper and more rusty and more mildewed in our West African backwater, as the Second Front opened in Europe with momentous confrontations. I was pleased to hear that my old ship, the *Rodney*, was in the thick of it, very successfully sending salvoes of its 16" shells seventeen miles inland to break up concentrations of German armour around Caen – the dear old, creaking lady was still stoutly earning her keep.

One of my more onerous duties was to be available (as PT Instructor, the 'Muscle Mechanic') to break up any fisticuffs likely to develop when the liberty boat came alongside with a load of drunken, aggressive sailors. There was a brand of beer, 'Black Horse', in the canteens and it truly was 'fighting beer'. Some great hairy Neanderthal Able Seaman would come up the gangway full of aggressive intent, looking to 'knock the PTI's block off', and the only successful gambit was to say, 'I'll come down to your mess in the morning and we'll have it out then.' Which I would, but by then he had sobered up and probably forgotten all about it. Good thing, he could easily have picked me up with one hand. But honour had been satisfied and the dignity of authority maintained.

There was another pleasant interlude. The Sergeants' Mess of the 3rd Sierra Leone Regiment invited a couple of us to have a ten-day spell ashore – and how luxurious that was after our rusty old bucket. We slept in comfortable beds with mosquito nets, were given a cup of tea by native servants on waking, fed like fighting cocks at breakfast, lunch and supper and were allowed to draw a .303 rifle and go hunting for bush fowl in the surrounding country. The bush fowl is a sort of West African partridge. We couldn't get them on the wing with a .303, which was like a sledgehammer to a nut, anyway, and it was a case of carefully stalking the timid, shy birds. Their meat was delicious.

There is not much else to tell about Freetown. All that remains in my recollection is the awful, never-ending, humid, enervating heat, the skin complaints like 'prickly heat' and the

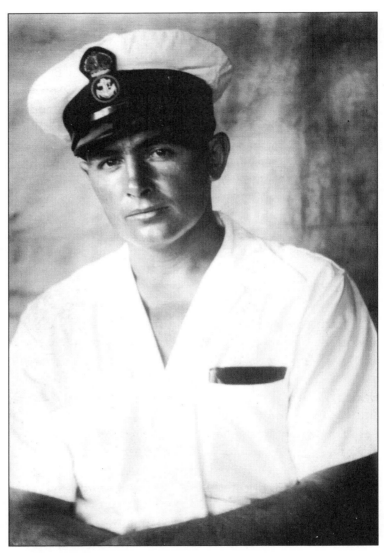

35. The author, Freetown, 1944.

yellow anti-malarial 'Mepacrine' tablets which, combined with our suntans, made us appear to have been steeped in extract of mahogany. Nothing lasts for ever and the humid months rolled slowly by until in May 1945 it was time to pack up one's gear and get on the boat for home. We looked across at her, anchored in the roads, the ship which was to take us to home and beauty – and she looked fantastic. Good riddance, we thought, as we got under way the next day and watched *Philoctetes* and the *Edinburgh Castle* diminish behind us. The only thing I can recall of the passage home was a U-boat scare on the last day, when we had already got into St George's Channel. The escort vessels did their thing and began tearing about and plastering the ocean with depth charges. Happily they scared off the U-boat and that was our last little patch of the War. Then we were alongside at Liverpool.

Within twenty-four hours the first lot (including me, praise be) were off the ship and making their way to Lime Street station for the train for Euston. Barbara met the train, looking just the sweet same. The main thing about that leave was that we decided to get married with the least delay. Even then, it was 21 July before we tied the knot, on my being allowed a further generous fortnight for the purpose.

CHAPTER IX

Naval Engineering

On reporting back in early July to HMS *Drake* the RN barracks in Devonport, I was posted to HMS *Thunderer*, the Royal Naval Engineering College, a shore-based school of engineering which had two branches. The oldest of these was within the dockyard perimeter at Keyham, Devonport, while the newer country branch had been established on the outskirts of Plymouth at Manadon, a landed estate of some antiquity with a fine old manor house, which comprised the headquarters offices, Captain's and officers' accommodation, wardroom and so on. The multitude of buildings comprising the engineering school were modern, light, airy and very pleasant to work in. The college also had a couple of light aircraft (Tiger Moths) out at a grass airfield at Roborough, some six miles from Plymouth on the road to Yelverton. 'Naval Engineering' perforce now included aeronautical engineering, by reason of the phenomenal growth and development in strength and importance of the Fleet Air Arm during the war years. Some of the Engineering Branch officers were qualified pilots, too, of course, including our Padre, who had a rich store of anecdotes of carrier warfare in the Pacific, alongside the Americans who were then fighting their way to Okinawa. I adroitly made sure the Padre was aware of my obsession with biplanes. On many occasions during rather empty forenoons, when the midshipmen were clossetted in the classrooms or the workshops, he would drop in to the gymnasium and suggest a flip over Plymouth Sound in a Tiger Moth. Happy mornings! We would pile into his little pre-war Austin Seven for the short ride to Roborough, find the aircraft readied, taxi to the end of the field and then up, up and away in the sunny Devon air, soaring over Plymouth Hoe which looked very grand from above. I loved those carefree mornings when we 'played hookey' (truanted) and enjoyed the summer day aloft. I expect it's virtually a metropolis down there now – I couldn't bear to go back and find my memories shattered. After all, it was fifty years ago.

After Freetown, the RNEC was a doddle, a very pleasant doddle. Apart from the old manor house, the Manadon branch consisted of living huts for the 'middies' in training, wonderfully equipped classrooms, engineering workshops, several good sports fields and a superb, spacious gymnasium, with a herringbone wooden block floor which must have cost a great deal of money. Near the workshops were several cavernous aircraft hangars, stuffed with the famous aircraft which had made such headlines over Britain, France, the Atlantic, Norway, Germany, Burma and the Pacific. I recall a Barracuda, Mosquito, Corsair, Swordfish (lovely aeroplane), Grumman Wildcat, Harvard, Albacore and Skua.

The 'middies' were given first-class hands-on training, which I doubt had an equal in the British Isles, in any commercial company. For two terms of the approximately four-year course, the midshipmen served on a training cruiser, getting seagoing experience of what their duties were really about. It was a good break for them and they saw something of the world early in their training. The PT Instructor on the training cruiser was one 'Ginger' Hobbs, a very dapper and 'all about' PTI who relished the pomp and circumstance and protocol of military life, and all the rest of military show. Whenever we met in the town he'd always salute my wife. On talking to a small group of the 'middies' who'd just returned from their sea terms, I asked them about Ginger Hobbs and how they had got on with him. They had enjoyed his instruction, apparently. I said, 'But he's full of flannel, you know.' 'Funny thing, Chief,' one of them mentioned. 'He said exactly the same thing about you!'

Some bright spark, no doubt imbued with the virtues of scrubbing the upper deck to make it look nice, organized the cleaners to give the gymnasium floor a jolly good slosh and a scrub. It looked beautifully clean for a little while, with a gratifying amount of dirt in the final rinsing water. Then it became alarmingly evident that the wooden blocks were beginning to absorb the water and swell. By the next morning it was not possible to walk on the floor at all. The previously flat gymnasium floor now resembled a very rough sea in the Bay of Biscay; and there were some very red faces. Our own programme of PT teaching was effectively fractured as were a host of other events and meetings for which the gym was used. It was some weeks before the floor was relaid, using the best of the old dried blocks and some painfully expensive new ones.

Before getting the train to London for my fortnight's leave to get married I paid a considerable sum, for those days, to a type of 'Interflora', or whatever it was called then, in Plymouth, for a bouquet of red roses to be delivered to Barbara before she left for the Register Office. Having previously got myself out of the house, I was standing in Streatham High Road when I saw Barbara's mother looking worried and carrying a limp and scrawny bunch of very tired flowers – these were the 'bouquet'. Prompt action was necessary. I said 'Leave it to me,' got a taxi to Moyses Stevens in Victoria, at the taxi driver's suggestion, beseeched them to make up a bouquet of red roses there and then, paid seven guineas for it, dived back into the taxi and delivered the flowers to Streatham on time – within the hour, in fact. As our small wedding group stood outside Wandsworth Register Office on that cloudy morning, the sun came out as the photographer took the pictures. A happy augury, a good omen . . . as it turned out. For forty-six years.

After a wedding lunch, Barbara and I departed for Waterloo Station, Guildford and the Orchard Farm Guest house, a few miles outside the town. We'd got instructions about the blue and red buses: 'Get the blue one from the station, then change at so-and-so for the red one. Get off the red bus at the potato patch and it's a short walk.' I was wearing some very good but stiff leather shoes I'd bought in Freetown; Barbara had dressed a little more sensibly. As it happened, the colours of the buses had recently been changed and the 'potato patch' was some one and a half square miles in extent. We had taken far too much luggage and had dismounted from the red bus at the wrong potato patch stop – about half a mile too early. It was quite a walk, with my shoes giving me hell. But the welcome at the guest house, some food and a bath soon turned it back into a honeymoon. There were no foreign trips and exotic destinations in those days. We were so happy we decided not to pursue the flower swindle. One of the guests was a

94-year-old lady who had been a missionary in Madagascar. She had some fascinating tales of times past, as we three sat under the apple tree in the garden. B and I used to go into Guildford to get things for her. This gracious, dignified and uncomplaining old lady had plainly been dumped in the guest house and conveniently forgotten. Life doesn't change.

Back at RNEC, the duties were anything but onerous. Perhaps the most demanding was getting out of the feathers in the early morning and mustering the middies outside one of the hangars for early morning exercises. I still wait to be convinced that this does anybody any good; health-wise, I mean. A little discomfort and inconvenience is good for the character, no doubt, but I never felt I was doing a large body of disgruntled and half-awake midshipmen any good by barking at them as the sun came up. I used to tease them a little bit. It was 1947 and the then Princess Elizabeth had just married Lieutenant Phillip Mountbatten RN. I said 'You will never grow up and marry a princess if you don't do your exercises, you know.' Humour at that hour of the morning was not well received, but it did liven them up a bit. There were no hard feelings. That evening, when we had the keen ones in the gymnasium to learn the rudiments of fencing, boxing and mat acrobatics, life was much more agreeable and things used to go with a swing.

Much of our time was taken up with refereeing football and rugger matches, arranging fixtures with opponents like the Camborne School of Mines in Cornwall, Tavistock School, Tiverton School and other good teams in the region. Once a year there was the Great Exeter to Plymouth Road Race. I forget now who we were running against, but the form was to pick a team of runners, who would cover the distance in relays, each running some five or six miles on the road from Exeter. A grand relay race, of course. The RNEC bus, carrying those who had completed their stint and those who had yet to run, followed the runners, stopping at each station on the way. I had, out of interest, completed a correspondence course on massage and was getting in some good practice on the aching legs of those whose stint had just been completed, as well as warming up those who had yet to run. I felt quite proud the year we won the race, because a report in the College magazine gave prominence to the reasons for our success – one of them being 'Petty Officer Grieve's patent embrocation in a Guinness bottle'.

On the Physical and Recreational Training strength were three – Lieutenant Nader, the P and RT Officer, RM Sergeant 'Wobbly' Mattson and myself (Fig. 36). 'Wobbly' had a most distinctive gait, characteristic of an old salt who'd never walked on anything but ship's decks, and in rough seas at that. When he rapped his knuckles on his cranium it really did sound as though he was knocking on wood – a favourite party trick. He was a great companion and a much-beloved chum. I was sad when he got posted elsewhere.

One of the most interesting features of being a staff member at the college was watching the midshipmen develop physically, and also in self-assurance and confidence. It was quite fascinating to observe boys becoming men, acquiring the capability of easy command as the months and years went by.

My interest in massage and allied therapies grew while I was at RNEC. 'Wobbly' and I purchased a simple radiant heat lamp and began 'treating', as best we knew how, joint strains and muscle pains. We had quite a little clinic

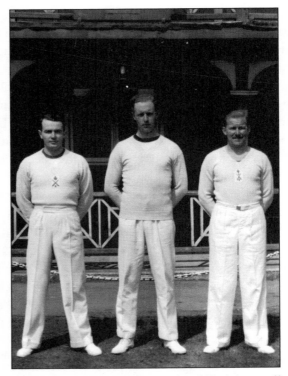

36. The Physical and Recreational Training staff
Royal Naval Engineering College, Devonport 1947.
From right to left: RM CSgt. Matson, Lt Nader, PO Grieve.

(unofficial) running in the gymnasium during the evenings and my interest we sufficiently stimulated to look further afield. In our training as PTIs we had received a certain amount of instruction in anatomy and physiology, and this was further developed in the correspondence massage course. I found the field immensely fascinating. Then I was invited to help, on one evening a week, at a private physiotherapy clinic in the town. It was mostly legwork, of course, but I did a lot of observing and learned a great deal which stood me in good stead later on – I noted who got better and who didn't, and on what treatment. Valuable early lessons. Inevitably, one saw that there was nothing for it but to do the full three-year training course of the Chartered Society of Physiotherapy. Since I was not in the 'Sick Berth' branch there was no hope that I might be sent for a CSP course while still in the service as a PTI.

In late 1947, Barbara retired from the Civil Service and came down to live with me in a reasonably priced flat. Service personnel were allowed, nay encouraged, to live ashore while serving in shore bases. She took a job in town and we set up our first ménage. Some days I'd even come home for lunch – the bus services were so reliable then – which often turned out to be beans on toast in Dingles, the department store, for ninepence (4p). She got a dowry, or a form of golden handshake, from the Civil Service and bought me a present – *Gray's Anatomy*, 29th Edition.

She, too, was beginning to perceive that a naval career was not for me. I'd got weary of the incessant foul language of ordinary conversation, and of not being able to choose the people I perforce had to live with. One could have tried for promotion to higher rank but I had had enough by then. It was something of a luxury to change horses in mid-stream, as it were, and had we started a family it would have been an irresponsible luxury. But our lives had been so disrupted by the War (which started when I was twenty-one, so I was twenty-seven when it ended) and the general murky outlook that a change of direction seemed as good a notion as any. I therefore began to consider the options as a civilian, since I had only a year left to serve. I would have to sign on for another ten years or take my discharge and my chance in civvy life. When only fifteen, in 1934, I'd had to sign on for 'twelve years from the age of 18' and in those days there was no hope of getting out of the service before one was thirty.

Barbara was the most unselfish woman in the world – I was a very fortunate man. She was quite content, enthusiastic even, that I should get a proper training, for what I wanted most in the world to do. Not knowing much of that field of work, in the great big world outside the protected cocoon of service life, the first thing would be to get a job, any job, and somewhere to live, and then plan from there. But for the moment that lay in the future. Meanwhile I had bought a hefty four-volume title: Watson-Jones's *Fractures and Joint Injuries*. I perceived that I would need to be well-versed in the area. Many would have said I was mad but I had got the bug by now. Without the basic requirements of a medical education, i.e. an introduction, I began to acquire a lot more information, all higgedly-piggedly in my mind but indisputably *there*. My mind began to bulge with the reading I was doing. I could not get enough of it. I soaked it up like a sponge. Soon I could rattle off the muscle attachments of the main groups like an old hand. I also began to perceive what a marvellous contraption was the human joint. Physiology (the *function* of the body) was a different matter. I had no guidance and did not know what I didn't know. Then I bought a physiology text and began to see in which direction I needed to expand my reading.

We made some good friends down there – now dead, alas. There was Nora, a local chiropodist, and her own friend and relation, Dr Sandy Vogler. He was one of the old school, a real live, old-fashioned General Practitioner, now near the end of his working life. He had some wonderful tales of his medical-student days at St Bartholomew's Hospital in London during the early years of the century. While B and I were awaiting the results of my final examinations, in May 1952, we rode our bone-shaker of a second-hand tandem (sans gears or any other modern gizmos) down to Plymouth to see our friends again – it took us three days. The first day we got as far as Ringwood, the next as far as Exeter and on the third day rode triumphantly into Plymouth – with sore backsides! B maintained she got more blisters on her heels from pushing the beast up hills than she did on her bum from riding it. We just couldn't face the return journey by tandem (gears would have made life easier) so went to North Road Station and asked how far our money would take us. 'Didcot' was the reply, so we loaded the tandem into the guard's van of this paper train and thankfully sank into seats more comfortable than the saddle of a second-hand tandem. We were turfed out at Didcot in the early hours of a lovely summer's day, and the ride home, through Pangbourne and some beautiful country, was a silent joy. Our machine made no noise and we saw red squirrels by the score and much other wildlife, as we sped along in silence. We were proud we'd got there, but would never have done it again. We arrived home to good news – I had passed my Finals examination.

One of the ship's cooks at RNEC was a keen boxing fan and eager to improve his skills at the fight game. He used to drop into the gymnasium when he was free and we would have a friendly sparring session. Although I had been a useful welterweight at the training establishment I was not a good boxer, being better at teaching it as a PTI than doing it for success. He began not pulling his punches as much as he should during our sparring and one day it got quite hot-tempered. It ended up with us having quite a set-to and after that the sparring sessions went out of the window.

Of much more interest were the evening sessions when we took a group of interested middies into the skills of fencing, with epée, sabre and foil. The last of these demanded the most skill and practice, and these fencing evenings were so much more interesting than heaving one's body about on the window bars, climbing ropes, parallel bars and leaping over box horses. On some early morning exercise I would take the assembled middies for a run, rather than a formal exercise period. We would trot round and behind the hangars, down to the sports field, back around the hangars and then into the gymnasium to finish. The wastage was alarming – one would start off with more than 300 young bodies and end up in the gymnasium with only 225 or so, the rest having simply disappeared off the face of the earth as we trotted around the hangars. It was best not to get too excited about 'dereliction of duty' but mentally to award marks for ingenuity and skilful skiving.

I haven't yet mentioned the PTI at the Keyham end – Chief Petty Officer Willie Sennett. He was just a natural-born fiddler, and whatever the circumstances Willie could see the potential of making a little profit on the side. When on some ship or other, he had got together a skilled water-polo team, and whenever the ship called at a likely port he would organize his team to go ashore in the usual way and then congregate with their gear at the local swimming bath. Willie had to cross the players' palms with silver, of course, but still made enough to make things well worth while. I'm sure it was in his genes, this extraordinary ability to get a profitable scam going out of the most unlikely circumstances. He, too, took the correspondence massage course, and had some business cards printed, anticipating his discharge from the Service. They read 'W. Sennett, Esq. Masseur and Fencing Master'. He's probably active in Heaven this very minute, flogging used wings at bargain prices to new entrants – and no questions asked. He was domiciled in Totnes and used to roar up there on his motorbike whenever he could. Where his petrol (strictly rationed) came from I have no idea.

During the late forties a New Zealand Navy cruiser came alongside in the dockyard and Willie was down there in a flash. Since he only had to go out of the back door of RNEC into the dockyard he thereby avoided any use of the official dockyard gates, guarded by the dockyard police who had authority to search all personnel and packages or goods passing through. Willie made a deal with the ship's tailor and had purchased a bolt of the best quality blue serge, which was soon smuggled into Keyham by the back door. Willie set up a thriving market among the WRNS and his colleagues, including me. I bought enough of the excellent material to make a snappy little blue serge suit for Barbara. Local dressmakers all over Devonport were suddenly very busy making blue serge suits for ladies.

Spontaneous testimonials are not easy to come by, which is why I enjoyed my visit to a destroyer in the dockyard. One of my shipmates had suggested I drop in to renew old memories, since we had been together in the *Norfolk* ten years before. There were three engineer officers attached to the destroyer for a few weeks, by reason of a new engine-room innovation under test, all of them 'old RNEC boys' from during my own time there. Nothing would do but for us to repair to the wardroom and get the gin out. They spoke of their RNEC time with affection, and apparently I had been more of a success than I had imagined. By the time I had got to the dockyard gate I was staggering a bit and seeing double. I spotted a group marching towards the gate so joined up with them and fell into step, since I did not want to be apprehended for being under the influence while in charge of a pair of shoes. I got through without incident and made it safely by bus back to RNEC and a short sleep in a corner of the gymnasium.

For some reason that I don't recall, I'd cooked up an inguinal hernia, which required surgical repair, and was admitted to the Royal Naval Hospital at Stonehouse, Devonport. A more important simultaneous event was the 1948 Olympic Games, which were held in London at Wembley Stadium. In those days it was customary to spend a long time in bed after simple operations like hernia repair and I was kept incarcerated for three weeks! I really began to get the idea I'd been through a major surgical procedure. Even four weeks afterwards I was still feeling I was fragile and taking great care of myself. I recall lying in bed and following the commentaries on the events from Wembley.

Time was passing and my fifteen years in the RN were nearly up. I expected Lieutenant Nader, the P and RT Officer, to summon me and point out the benefits of staying in the service for another ten years, which he did. To no avail; I was dying to be off and away and free of the Navy at last. Barbara turned her job in, we paid the final week's rent for the flat, packed up our few possessions in a tea chest, sent it on ahead, had a small farewell party at RNEC and got the train for London. I had to go to Woking, if I recall, to collect my 'demob' suit and other bits and pieces of my government-issue civilian outfit, none of which gave one much confidence in one's appearance. The collection even included cheap cuff-links and collar studs, so was nominally complete. I sold the lot for two pounds within a week. The snag was that all the best gear had been picked out by my predecessors during the previous two years. I enjoyed being a civilian drone during the period of my demob leave and then got a job, at five pounds a week, as a production control clerk in a board and packaging mill at Tooting, London SW17. To this day I have no idea what it was I was supposed to be controlling but I'd made it. I was out of the Navy and I'd got a job. It was a strange time and the future looked very uncertain. By dint of walking around Streatham and keeping my eyes open, I found a comfortable and reasonably priced flat. I'd been given a gratuity of £98.00 and with other resources we bought dining room and bedroom suites and moved in. We had reached a crossroad and I'm still not sure, fifty years later, whether we did the right thing or not.

CHAPTER X

The Physiotherapist

I was full of aspiration to qualify as a physiotherapist, and on my bus journeys from Streatham to Tooting and back used to daydream of helping to make better patients with musculo-skeletal problems, children with poliomyelitis (infantile paralysis), men and women with respiratory difficulties, athletic strains and sprains and all the other myriad conditions which I knew could be helped by good physiotherapy. I was so mesmerized by my Holy Grail that I didn't stop to consider the significance of our ages. I was thirty and Barbara thirty-two, and on qualification I'd be thirty-three and she thirty-five. Simple qualification did not make a physiotherapist. There followed the exacting pursuit of clinical experience in general work, orthopaedics, paediatrics, neurology, respiratory conditions, chest surgery and so on. I'd be forty before I'd realized my aim of comprehensive clinical experience and Barbara would be forty-two – not the best time to start a family. I wish I had known then what I knew later, but don't we all. We spend our lives learning how to live and by the time we know all the answers it's too late and we are too old. Present opportunities have been missed because we fix our eyes on distant peaks and cannot see what is at our feet. In the 4th century BC, Mencius wrote: 'The path of duty lies in what is near, yet man seeks for it in what is remote.' I felt I had so much to catch up on – so much to repair of the largely barren wasted years in the Navy. I wanted to develop myself more fully, to become a more complete person before starting a family, because I didn't feel ready. Foolish mistake. This wrong-headed approach to life is well expressed by José Ortega Y Gasset: 'We cannot put off living until we are ready. The most salient characteristic of life is its coerciveness, its immediacy; it is always urgent – here and now – without any possible postponement. Life is fired at us point-blank.' I should not have hesitated on the brink, I should have jumped and grown wings to fly with on the way down. But I did not – I began to beaver away at my books like a maniac with a terrible obsession. We should have started a family then, and by coping with the difficulties would have grown up. But we (I) did not.

I digress for a moment now. Two or three years before she died in 1991 Barbara, now a 73-year-old below-knee amputee, sat in the car while I did some errand or other. She observed on the pavement nearby a mother and her young daughter, and she marked the unique rapport, the loving bond between them, manifest in the way they each doted on the beloved object, looking at each other with love in their eyes. When we got home Barbara described what she had perceived, and then said, in a quiet voice of infinite regret, 'I never had that.' It pierced my heart – I felt a great sadness, a terrible guilt, and a deep anger that we had both given so much of ourselves, our time, our lives and our energies to the dispensing and teaching of good physiotherapy. I know that I shall feel that deep remorse, that bitter regret, to the end of my days. But it is too late now and I must swallow the bitter pill. I could, like the schoolmaster in *Goodbye Mr Chips*, say 'Barbara and I have got *thousands* of children, all over the world' since I have taught many thousands either directly or through my books and tape-slide programmes, but she never had the feeling of her own child in her arms, and I devoutly wish I had given her that, at least. She gave me so much. There remains a certain sense of achievement, but at its centre is the feeling that it was at her expense.

We were both proud of what we had achieved, as a pair of starry-eyed idealistic amateurs who were quite prepared to work all hours, but I am now left with only negative emotions.

But back in January 1949 Barbara, as one of the most unselfish women in the world, took the line 'If that is what you want to do, so be it, that is what we do.' I applied to the Chartered Society of Physiotherapy for details of training, sat an entry examination which I sailed through, got a grant from the London County Council of £2.00 a week, turned in my job at Tooting and started training at the Field and Morris School of Physiotherapy, Albany Terrace, London NW1. Barbara supported me to the hilt, got an administrative job locally at £5.00 a week and we were away, doing what I wanted to do. One of the Society's requirements was that I study chemistry and physics for six months, concurrently with my training, since my education in that direction was lacking. I always did lean to arts rather than science, but once I got my teeth into the basics of science I was away. I used to cycle from the Great Portland Street area of London (near the physiotherapy school) to the Working Men's College in Crowndale Road, Camden, on several evenings a week, trying to grasp the elements of chemistry and physics after a day's work at the school. Then I would cycle home from Camden to Streatham, from NW1 to SW16, a considerable distance. My classmates were in the 18-22 age range, many of them with matriculation and university-entrance equivalents, and initially they scared the living daylight out of me. How on earth am I going to keep up with this lot? I wondered. Their casual approach to education puzzled me, since I was only too grateful for being given the chance to train. I valued every scrap of information, devoured every book that came my way, queried everything I was not sure of. I bought a pocket Medical Dictionary and devoured that, too. I soon began to perceive that I was better placed than they were. I was more experienced in life after fifteen years in the Navy, I'd done some living and had also seen a fair bit of dying during the War. I was not keen on socializing and kicking my heels up – I'd already done that, too. I was relatively mature, very happily married with a secure, loving home life and had no distractions to tempt me away from my dedicated pursuit of *everything* to do with physiotherapy and allied subjects. Also, I had begun to note that I was good at soaking up knowledge and slotting each new accretion into a logical storage plan in my mind, and also good at expressing myself on paper – a nasty little swot with the gift of the gab, some may say. Whatever it was (is), it stood me in good stead. I was able, as time went by, to see that some of the textbooks we used were not all that well put together. Definitions were imprecise and textual material not well organized. I began to feel I could at least do as well if not better, and secretly nurtured the intention, when my experience was wider and complete, to have a go at producing my own textbooks. But that lay some forty years in the future.

The supply of physiotherapy teachers was neither regular nor of consistent quality. One or two were outstanding, as exemplified by James Guest who taught me so much as a student and who was later my Principal when I joined the teaching staff of his school at the West Middlesex Hospital in Isleworth. Also Miss Hazel Stannard, whose teaching of the small muscles of the hand and the foot have remained with me to this day. Some of the 'teachers' were quite hopeless and just made everybody angry. At one stage, I got so fed up with the sloppy teaching that I purchased a copy of the syllabus from the Chartered Society, for one shilling, and decided to work my way through it on my own, from A to Z, regardless of the stage of teaching I was being subjected to at the school.

It was at times a rough and lonely furrow to plough, but I was gaining the sure knowledge that I had covered every single square centimetre of the ground. My success in the Preliminary Examinations (Anatomy and Physiology) strengthened my resolve. I got a Credit in that examination, and in the Intermediate and Final Examinations, too, and in fact came top of my year in the whole country, winning the Manley Memorial Prize. Not bad for someone who left school at fourteen. Much of life in the decade after the War was like that – hand to mouth. Bread rationing continued after the War, as did clothes rationing. It was a long and weary time before austerity and difficulty and shortages gave way to easement and plenty – for most of us, anyway.

There was little or no money for books. I would occasionally get good second-hand ones from Foyle's in Charing Cross Road, and another recourse was Marylebone Library, a magnificent establishment just down the road from the school. On days euphemistically devoted to 'Free Study', i.e. no teacher available, I would walk down to the library and bury my head in their treasures. It is no exaggeration to say that I learned almost all of my 'General Pathology' in Marylebone Library. I soaked up so much knowledge in that august establishment I'd like to give it a large gold medal. Of special value was Dible and Davies's *Pathology*, a tome which gave me so much to think about. I also applied to the SSAFI – the Soldiers', Sailors' and Air Force Institute – in the Brompton Road, Knightsbridge, for a grant to buy books. My temerity paid off and I was given the princely sum of ten pounds, upon which I shot off to the Charing Cross Road and Foyle's Medical Section. It was in the Marylebone Library that I perceived how many of the classical old medical texts were literature, too. In times past doctors were learned and erudite philosophers also, and well-versed in the business of expressing themselves with precision, economy and style.

The London postal district NW1, and the Regent's Park area generally, have always had great significance for me. It was the site of the Physiotherapy School, of Park Village East where we lived for four and a half years; it was also the stamping ground of the turn-of-the century painters whose work I loved – Gore, Gilman, Sickert and others of the London Group, and it was close to the Royal National Orthopaedic Hospital, in Great Portland Street, where I worked for four and a half happy years. Regent's Park, and the zoo, were early fixed in my mind when, in 1926, we were taken to see the elephants and I remarked 'Hark at the smell.' No. 8 Fitzroy Street was the site of Sickert's studio, and some fifty yards from our flat in Park Village East was Granby Street, where Sickert painted so many of his beautiful *contre jour* nudes. Then there was Camden High Street; there is *nothing* which cannot be obtained in Camden High Street and its environs. The cosmopolitan, polyglot crowds of Camden High Street were only a stone's throw from the stately Nash terraces of Regent's Park, and only a further stone's thrown from Harley Street, Cavendish Street and Weymouth Street. A lovely, distinctive and aristocratic part of London.

An essential part of our training was familiarization with the ordinary duties and running of a hospital ward. My initiation into this medical hewing of wood and drawing of water took place in the Children's Ward of the Royal Waterloo Hospital, at the southern end of Westminster Bridge. I carried the little patients about, made them comfortable, took temperatures and handled their bottles and potties. I once had this angelic small boy, with lovely saucer eyes of the deepest blue, sitting on my lap and opening his mouth at regular intervals for me to shovel some more in. Then it became plain that he had opened the other end, too, and was now sporting an expression which plainly said, 'Aren't I clever? Doing all that at the same time?' I had a rather noisome ride home on my bicycle.

The hospital is now defunct, I believe.

I didn't always spend 'Free Study' time in Marylebone Library. There was a good newsreel cinema at Baker Street, and my student chum Ben Davies and I used to go there to see films of the latest fights. It was there we saw the famous World Middleweight Title fight between Randolph Turpin and Sugar Ray Robinson, which Turpin won, only to lose it again in New York a few months later. Thereafter, when finances allowed, I used to go to Earl's Court or Haringay to see the prominent fighters of the day in action. My companion then was Steve Donovan, a fellow student and also a jazz guitarist, who played with the best of the leading bands of the day. He lived in a flat in Victoria with two doctors who specialized in Physical Medicine. One of them, Dr Ivor Contran, worked at St Thomas's Hospital, just across the river from the Houses of Parliament. This was a happy coincidence for me, since while still in the Navy I had bought an eye-opener of a book, *Deep Massage and Manipulation Illustrated* by Dr John Carfax, who was then one of the Consultants in Physical Medicine at St Thomas's Hospital. I had devoured the book before I left the Navy and had begun to see the way I wanted to go, i.e. specialization in 'Joint Manipulation'. There was already a history of manipulation being taught at STH – in earlier years by Dr J.B. Marlowe, who wrote several classic texts on the subject. During holidays between terms at the Physiotherapy School, I got permission, by the kind intercession of Dr Conran, to just stand around and watch the treatments on the clinical shop floor at STH. I was all eyes, ears and wits – everything wide open to soak up all I could about this fascinating speciality, which seemed to me to directly address so many of the common muscular and joint aches and pains afflicting so many. Dr Carfax revolutionized Physical Medicine by his original thinking and new approach to old problems. He trained very many thousands of therapists worldwide, by his presence, his teaching, that of his disciples and his books, which have gone into dozens of editions and reprints. A very great deal of what physiotherapists do today has developed from his original work during the forties. We all owe him so much. It was my special pleasure to write a seventieth birthday tribute to him in our journal. While I took every opportunity to further my interest in this speciality, I was steadily getting through my training. Some two and a half years after commencing at the school we took our Intermediate Examinations. By this time the work seemed just cherry pie to me and I was able to apply much of my earlier physical training in the Royal Navy. Six months later we took our Finals – by this time I did not need to cycle miles and miles all over London. I spent my time in the Physical Medicine Departments of hospitals, as though a member of the staff – under supervision.

It was a while waiting for the final results that B and I cycled to Plymouth on an old tandem, described on page 191. Soon after that I was a qualified but inexperienced physiotherapist. While in Plymouth I had looked in on an exhibition of paintings by Bernard Dunstan – it was love at first sight. There were some truly beautiful things, at prices like £25 each, which was an astronomical sum for me in those days. Would that I could see those paintings and those prices again now. I would have bought the lot. Dunstan wrote some very useful books, including a handful for the self-taught amateur, and in later years I gained immensely from his teaching of my other love – painting in oils.

In May 1952, there began the exacting pursuit of clinical experience, which began with a year's general work at the Miller General Hospital in Greenwich, a part of London which (then) had seen better days and still retained strong links with the Royal Navy and Merchant Marine. It seems a century ago now. One got a 109 bus from Streatham to Kennington Oval, and then a 163 tram which used to wallow and trundle all the way east through Peckham, Camberwell

204

and Deptford to Greenwich. Physiotherapy jobs were not all that easy to come by in 1952 and the Miller General was the nearest I could get to Streatham. While serving on the staff there I was informed I had won the Manley Memorial Prize, for the top student of my year. I felt so proud when it was presented to me at the 1953 Physiotherapy Congress, held in the Westminster Hall, London, by Professor Willis. He was one of the Editors of *Gray's Anatomy*, 29th Edition, no less, the one Barbara 'stood' me in Plymouth in 1947.

Soon it was time to move on again, and in 1953 I began work at the Queen Mary's Hospital for Children at Carshalton, in Surrey. While the children were the merriest bunch one could come across, it was nevertheless a sad place. So many young lives, blighted by tuberculosis of joints (usually spines and hips), infantile paralysis, talipes equino-varus (club foot), myasthenia gravis (a progressive weakening of muscle) and the various types of muscular dystrophy. There was a whole ward full of boys with muscular dystrophy, wards full of poliomyelitis (infantile paralysis) and wards full of tuberculous joints. The last were treated by the sanatorium principle of the day – lots of rest in the open air, often for a year or more. The children lay on spinal carriages or other frames in rows outside, covered by tarpaulins if the weather was wet and given extra blankets when it was cold. They became remarkably hardy, and only in the severest weather were they brought in under the verandah, still open on one side to the rain and snow. It was quite extraordinary how they remained mischievous and cheerful under the most strict of open-air treatment regimes. So far as tuberculosis was concerned, both the treatment and the outlook of these young people improved enormously on the advent of three drugs, most effective when given in combination – streptomycin, isoniazid and para-aminosalicylic acid. No doubt things have moved on since those days, yet tuberculosis is on the increase again and the too liberal use of antibiotics in other spheres of medicine have encouraged the emergence of super-bugs which seem to thrive on antibiotics for breakfast, as it were. It was sad to go onto the wards full of polio and to note the wasted limbs and soft-tissue contractures (shortening) of angelic small children. The treatment regime was that devised by Sister Kenny, in that as soon as practicable splints were discarded for the most part, in favour of muscle stretching, postural correction, training in correct walking patterns and strengthening of muscle, so far as that was possible. The children were brought down to the physiotherapy department on trolleys, and placed in hot baths to soak – this softened up the tissues and made stretching easier and more effective. There usually followed some hanky panky with a hose, which the children adored. They were then wrapped in enormous towels, placed on waist-high tables and subjected to a careful and meticulous drill of tissue stretching. Contracture (tissue shortening) was a disaster for the polio child, perhaps even more so than muscle weakness.

It was gratifying to note the circulation in their limbs improving, with dry, scaly skin becoming soft, supple, pink and healthy. Many of the children were helped by corrective surgery, but there was always some residual defect, of course. Like the advent of the anti-TB drugs, the Salk vaccine for polio was a major medical advance, on a par with the eradication of smallpox.

* * *

It was now 1954, and time to change again. I'd had no experience of working on surgical chest wards, and great things were going on in thoracic medicine and surgery which I wanted to know about. As soon as I spotted a vacancy at the London Chest Hospital, Victoria Park, East London I applied for the job. It was quite a journey – a 137 bus from Streatham, then change onto the Underground somewhere in the City for Bethnal Green, deep in the East End. Having got the job I was given the obligatory Mantoux Test, i.e. an inoculation of highly diluted 'Old Tuberculin' into the skin. The test should provoke a mild, localized reaction, which denotes the presence of antibodies from a previous subclinical (and therefore unnoticed) infection which has been recovered from. If the test is negative in adults, it usually indicates an absence of previous infection and therefore a lack of immunity, the person thus being unsuitable for employment in sanatoria or other establishments treating tuberculosis. I had quite a reaction, including a grandiose and thumping headache of quite hideous intensity. I have a clear recollection of walking home from the hospital to Bethnal Green Underground station and trying to glide along the pavement, since the slightest jar of each step viciously provoked my head pain. Being banged about on the Underground and jolted on the long bus-ride home nearly did for me that day. Most of the operations were for tumours of the lung or bronchus, and tuberculosis, with a host of ancillary or minor procedures in which physiotherapy played no great part, other than a check and correction of breathing patterns. The operation of thoracoplasty, in which ribs are removed and/or shortened, to collapse the lung and therefore rest it, were beginning to be phased out and I saw little of them. It was a three-stage procedure, with each of the stages separated by three weeks or so, and the patients needed a large dose of fortitude and durability to go through with it. Yet before the advent of effective drug therapy, it was often the only step left and did bring recovery to many tuberculosis victims who had otherwise reached the end of the road. The gross disturbance of thoracic architecture, by removal of ribs, profoundly disturbed spinal posture too, and until corrective physiotherapy was instituted some horrendous trunk deformities occurred. There were some very skilled therapists working in thoracic surgery in those days, and some highly effective teamwork between surgeons, nursing staff and physiotherapists.

But my heart remained in the manual treatment of common spinal 'musculoskeletal' conditions and I was over the moon when I received an invitation to join the staff at St Thomas's Hospital, in Dr Carfax's department. I jumped at it, and so left behind the world of thoracic medicine and surgery, in May 1955. Yet I was a better physiotherapist for the experience.

I also enjoyed the now simple journey – a single bus ride from Streatham to Lambeth. One felt very much in the central area of London, working just across the river from the Houses of Parliament, between Lambeth and Westminster bridges, close to Waterloo Station, near the Tate Gallery and not far from the South Bank and the Festival Hall. I felt honoured to became part of Florence Nightingale's old hospital and began to walk an inch or two taller. There was only one other male incumbent, Anthony Phillips, among the host of female physiotherapists. He could have fiercely resented the advent of another man, yet could not have been kinder or more welcoming. At coffee-time in the forenoons he would appear at the door of my section and jerk his head in the direction of the cafeteria. I learned a very great deal from Tony, who'd been doing manipulative work there for some years before I joined the staff. He did sterling work in clinical teaching of the candidates on the long post-registration Manipulation courses. After I had left STH, I used to arrange for the course students to sit in on Dr Carfax's clinics and then to hear a lecture from Anthony. I hope he is still alive and well.

Conscious of my good fortune, I immersed myself in the management of musculoskeletal conditions of the spine and limbs. Having bought the books of Dr J.B. Marlowe, Dr Carfax's predecessor (one of them while I was still in the Navy) and those of Dr Carfax, too, I applied myself to their thorough digestion on the home ground, as it were. It became plain to me even then that there was some dichotomy, some difference of concept and handling of these common aches and pains. While Dr Marlowe's approach of precision and gentleness was akin to osteopathic philosophy, Dr Carfax's method was original and distinctive. He considered the intervertebral disc to be involved in most cases of benign spinal pain, and his teaching on the sacro-iliac joint, for example, differed from that of Dr Marlowe. The manipulative techniques and explanations of their effect also differed. These differences of approach, technique and rationale were just a microcosm of what we still see today, worldwide. Several disparate groups of clinical workers, each in their own clinical discipline, are handling the same spinal and peripheral joint and soft tissue problems in disparate ways, yet each is still getting enough patients better to stay

interesting and a little less stark. In like manner, a prodigious
volume of research, especially in the Antipodes, has been
completed over the last three decades by physiotherapists,
and recognized worldwide. Physiotherapists have made a
significant contribution to the way we now think about these
common problems, and to our therapeutic successes.

I was fortunate enough to learn a very great deal at St
Thomas's Hospital from Dr Carfax and shall always be
grateful for it. Yet I began to find the Carfax idiom something
of a straightjacket and just had to spread my wings and think
for myself. Of particular value was the STH system of
continuing clinical assessment during treatment, so much so
that this philosophy is now firmly embedded in manipulative
practice across the world. I also learned much from Dr Alan
Southard who had a foot in both camps, as an experienced
osteopath and Consultant in Physical Medicine to the Brook
Hospital, Shooter's Hill, London S.E.

In 1958, after I had completed some three and a half years
at STH, one of the staff physicians was appointed Consultant
Rheumatologist at St Nicholas's Hospital, Plumstead, in East
London, and suggested I apply for the vacant post of
Superintendent Physiotherapist there. While I did not relish a
twice-daily drive of thirteen miles through the thick of
London rush-hour traffic it was a step up – so I applied and
was appointed. I learned there that I am no administrator. I
love to get my hands on problems and was quite hopeless at
delegating. To put it plainly, I was not a success, and things
were not helped by my growing inclination to begin teaching
my special interest to others. One of the more positive aspects
of my time as an unsatisfactory Superintendent was the
beginning of a durable friendship with two members of the

staff – JC and FH – with whom I am still in pleasurable contact. Both are now in Vancouver, one of them since retired. Down the years since then, JC and I have collaborated in a great many enterprises, e.g. a demonstration of lifting and handling techniques at the Friend's House in Euston Road, the proposal and founding of a Manipulation Association of Chartered Physiotherapists, together with another colleague (JJ), the formulation of an MACP Tape and Film Library, frequent practice sessions at JJ's private clinic in Devonshire Street, London, and innumerable other MACP alternatives, including much 'hands-on' teaching.

After a little more than two years as an indifferent Superintendent, there was nothing for it but to go back to STH to become a trainee teacher – another two years of anatomy to higher standard, likewise physiology, and the theory and practice of teaching. The physiotherapy students were most indulgent of my efforts, and one group even gave me a pewter tankard on my leaving as a fully fledged teacher.

A discipline which taught me much about organizing my own information was to have to prepare each of my lectures for perusal by one or other of the senior teachers. At first I considered their strictures to be quite merciless and unfair, yet soon began to perceive that they were steadily making me better at it; until I had reached the stage where every single possible loophole inviting stricture had been closed by meticulous and comprehensive preparation. Another golden lesson, very quickly and painfully learned, was never, ever, to go in front of a class without the most thorough preparation. A third, and equally painful lesson, was the realization that every group of young people, students, always included one

in business. Thus physical medicine, rheumatology, orthopaedic medicine, physiotherapy, osteopathy, chiropractic,
naturopathy and bone-setters (archaic term) are just names
for the great constellation of clinical workers and disciplines,
some orthodox and some lay, engaged in this field of work.
We see it in religion and concepts of spirituality, too, and
have only to consider Christianity, Buddhism, Catholicism,
Islam, Scientology, Shintoism and so on, to note the same
fracturing of human endeavour, aspirations, concepts of
heaven and hell, and spirituality. We sorely need a therapists'
Ecumenical Council of some kind, because the fiercely
partisan approach of many clinical workers, the posturing
and the strident claims that 'We are the only way, the truth
and the light' are just silly. While each may have their
preferred line of country, it must be recognized that the other
fellow and his lot may also have got a bit of the truth.

I began to get, and to expand, my intellectual bearings at
STH on a scale I never did elsewhere. To be wholly
concerned on the clinical shop floor with the work which
interested me most, and to be able to question at first hand
the authors of the books I used for guidance, was an
opportunity I took with both hands. Once I knew enough to
make comparisons and a choice, my own approach began to
include the osteopathic concept to a degree, since that
discipline (though osteopathy is a meaningless word)
recognizes the need for gentle, persuasive repetitious
movements as well as the brisk manipulative thrust. Since
those days of much clinical heart-searching about the best
procedures, there have evolved a multitude of different
approaches, a variety of techniques without hazard, which
have made life on the clinical shop floor vastly more

or more 'Clever Dicks'. It took me some time to devise my own strategy, which was simply to say, 'And by the way, Miss ... or Mr ... please remember that nobody loves a smart-arse', delivered quietly and almost as an afterthought. One also quickly learned the strategy of anticipating likely questions, and having to hand an answer for each one. An additional golden lesson was that there is no shame in admitting 'I don't know,' since students appreciate and respond to honesty. Neither students nor children are ever really fooled – they are quick to recognize the false front. It is always much easier and more relaxing to start a discussion as to where the answer to the question might be found. A further lesson for me was that if you embark on the teaching of children and/or students, by them you will be taught; and the final lesson for me at least, was that to teach well one must give it heart, soul, mind, body, blood and whatever else one has got. I do not believe that there is any such animal as an effective half-hearted teacher. It pressed me to the top of my bent, but it was just lovely to hear the metaphorical penny drop – to see the dawning of understanding of a new proposition, on the young faces, to get the considered answer to a question, which could only have been arrived at by constructive thought applying the principles already given.

It took me a long time to master the art of guiding the young students towards answers by encouraging their own reasoning abilities. There is not much of this in the early teaching of anatomy, but even in that case it is possible to slowly reveal the rightness and biomechanical sense behind the structure of a muscle and its function, or the attachments of an important ligament.

Physiology lends itself earlier to reasoning, which becomes

more exciting and absorbing as one grasps the beauty of the body's functions.

During the two years of my teacher training (1961-3) an Australian physiotherapist, Geoffrey Moorland, visited St Thomas's Hospital, since by this time it was an internationally known Physical Medicine Department where the students were taught joint manipulation as an integral part of physiotherapy. Moorland already had a foot in England, since he came here to do his bit during the War, much of which he spent flying Short Sunderland flying boats of Coastal Command from Pembroke Dock in Wales. I should mention here that Moorland had read very extensively, and was familiar with the writings and clinical idiom of many of the internationally known workers in this field, particularly Fryette, Southard, Carfax and both J.B. Marlowe and his son J.M. Marlowe. At that time Moorland had devised his own distinctive and graded approach to joint problems – more correctly neuro-musculo-skeletal problems – and was prepared to go to the trouble of looking at the work of others so that he might evaluate his own standing, worldwide, in the field. I have the feeling that his sojourn strengthened his sense of his own worth and gave him confidence to follow his own star.

He was at STH for some weeks, and I always found him ready to listen to others before expounding his own views. What was especially noticeable about his techniques was their graded gentleness and extreme precision. Accurate and meaningful diagnosis of these conditions is notoriously difficult, and rather than ascribe most benign spinal pain to abnormalities of the intervertebral disc, Moorland would suggest 'I don't know what the diagnosis is, but what I am treating is the pain.' He was not afraid to suggest that one frequently got the patient better without ever really knowing what the patient had got! This is not as daft as it sounds. If patients do not die of benign joint and soft-tissue pains, and therefore do not undergo post-mortem to discover what killed them, it is sometimes anybody's guess as to what the trouble was. Soothing terms like 'fibrositis', 'slipped disc', 'pulled muscle', 'pulled ligament', 'joint derangement' and so on may indeed be true, but it is very difficult to be sure. There is also the light-hearted approach of so long as you get them better without delay you can call it what you like, since nobody but the Almighty *really* knows and He's not talking. I exaggerate a little – we are now more aware of a proportion of these diagnoses, but the extent of our ignorance exceeds that of our certain knowledge.

Besides visiting STH, Moorland went to other centres in the UK and also to the USA, to visit Dr J.M. Marlowe, the physician son of Dr J.B. Marlowe, Dr Carfax's predecessor at STH. The younger Dr Marlowe was then working at a College of Osteopathic Medicine in the state of Michigan, USA.

Moorland and and I perceived an affinity between us, and it was the beginning of an association, sometimes stormy, which was to last for over thirty-five years – with pleasure and profit on both sides. We both had the pleasure, with other physiotherapists, of mounting post-registration, now post-graduate, manipulation courses of increasing standard and length – he in Adelaide, South Australia and me in London at the West Middlesex Hospital, Isleworth. Both courses began initially in 1965. It was at this hospital that I began my teaching career, under the principalship of my old teacher of student days, the estimable James Guest. It was just like old times to be under his wing again.

Barbara and I began to find the pace a little too hot, and longed to get out of London for a breather. Having toured Suffolk in 1958, when we became enchanted with its quiet beauty, its wide and lonely estuaries and its natives, all of whom seemed, after London, to be in possession of their own souls, we decided to seek a house up there. We found one in 1964, a pair of sound cottages, a 'double dweller', on a south-facing slope of one acre at Cratfield, about halfway between Ipswich and Norwich. The cottages, originally oak and plaster, were brick-walled, had sound roofs, water and electricity, although one was uninhabitable pending refurbishment. The freehold price was £1,000. When other demands permitted, we used to pile into the car, loaded with bricks, cement, wood, screws etc., after work on a Friday and drive up to Suffolk, turn in at once and get cracking on the 'do-it-yourself' for one and a half days, before going home at midday on the Sunday so that Barbara could do the week's washing and I could prepare the teaching for the next week. It might be said we were out of our tiny minds, but Cratfield gave us so much pleasure. There was a lovely thirties feel about the place and the people then. Eventually we moved to Suffolk for good and had many lovely years together in that sweet place. We sold the cottages for £16,500 in 1975, and had some change left after buying a commodious Edwardian bungalow ('Hill Drive') in about three quarters of an acre in Halesworth, the nearest town.

CHAPTER XI

Developing the Speciality

As my clinical involvement in the manipulation scene, both as teacher and practitioner, hotted up during the mid-sixties, so one was invited to travel further afield, teaching here, there and everywhere. In the decade 1965-75, there was hardly a big town in mainland Britain that I hadn't visited on a teaching assignment. These trips were in addition to the long courses for the Chartered Society of Physiotherapy, which were initially mounted by myself and one of Dr Carfax's physiotherapists, Miss Janet Hayling, at the West Middlesex Hospital. Geoff Moorland came to England again in 1966, and joined the duo of Miss Hayling and me at WMH, to provide two courses during that year. I recall a particularly successful one he held at the Westminster Hospital, just up the road from the Tate Gallery, on the north side of the river. These were often weekend introductory courses, or a course spread over six to eight weeks, two days a week. Often a weekend would be devoted to a particular joint, e.g. the elbow, the cranio-spinal junction, sacro-iliac joint or the jaw joints. The pace was so hectic, and the days so full, that I have only the most vague recollection of where I taught and precisely what I did during that, for me, explosive decade.

217

We also organized monthly meetings of the Manipulation Association, as well as courses for the Organisation of Chartered Physiotherapists in Private Practice. I began to find the demand of teaching general physiotherapy, as well as fostering so much involvement in manipulative treatment, a bit too much for me. I was also producing a newsletter every two months, which Barbara enthusiastically typed and distributed worldwide, and I was beginning to plan a small paperback book for beginners. It became necessary to envisage a specialist teaching post, based at one or other hospital, to which candidates would be attracted as to a centre. In other words, a Physiotherapists' Manipulation School. After enquiries, the Consultant Rheumatologist (Dr Brookes) at Oldchurch Hospital in Romford, Essex, offered to try and establish an officially-sponsored Post-Registration Teaching Centre. Taking my life in my hands, as it were, I bade farewell to my old alma mater (the West Middlesex Hospital) and shifted lock, stock and barrel to Romford. Barbara and I found a suitable flat nearby and she was transferred from London SW16 to the Romford Branch of Brooke Street Bureau, for whom she was then working. I had accepted a drop in salary from that of a teacher with six years' seniority to that of a senior physiotherapist.

I began to breathe the sweet air of clinical freedom, and could forget all about forms of physiotherapy other than that of my clinical interest. A nice feeling, but at some cost. I organized three long annual courses, those of 1970, 1971 and 1972. Practical and written examinations were held at the end of each course as the comprehensiveness of the teaching gradually increased. It was always a slog, but I gloried in it and enjoyed the teaching. Yet the stark fact was that I had no formal copper-bottomed recognition of what I was doing. I was still running at a financial loss and only by the good fortune of having a devoted wife was I able to operate at all.

We stuck this for two and a bit more years, when it became obvious that Dr Brookes's ducks were swans, and that his plans were a little more difficult to realize than he had imagined. Barbara and I decided we had given enough to physiotherapy and the manipulation cause, and were seriously considering getting out of physiotherapy altogether and starting a new life in Suffolk selling seeds. Then completely out of the blue I received an invitation to set up a teaching unit at the Royal National Orthopaedic Hospital in Great Portland Street, W1. This was more like it. The charm of the new proposal was that it would be a specialist unit, with the use of an excellent lecture theatre, and I would receive a Vice-Principal's salary. I jumped at it. We found a good flat in Park Village East, just up Albany Street from the hospital, and Barbara obtained a good and promising post at the Medical Research Council, close by at Park Crescent, W1. Here we were back once more in the Regent's Park area of London and full of joy at the prospect.

We were still spending many weekends travelling here, there and everywhere teaching. I cannot remember even half of the hospitals we visited, but do recall among others Swansea, Bristol, Manchester, Canterbury, Leeds, St Andrews, Orpington, Sheffield, Worthing, Liverpool, Norwich and Oxford. Superintendents of Departments, teachers and even Principals of Schools were beginning to apply for the long courses, which had begun to expand out of all recognition. Happily, I had been chosen to lecture at the 1974 World Congress for Physical Therapy in Montreal, and could thus be present at the Inauguration of the International Federation of Orthopaedic Manipulative Therapists. This was the culmination of our earlier tentative deliberations at the 1970 WCPT in Amsterdam. I had produced a little paperback, merely a reproduction of Barbara's typed pages, on essential basics for the beginner, and took a bundle of them to the subsequent meeting of the IFOMT, in 1975, in the Canary Islands. They sold like hot cakes – an encouragement.

I digress for a little while. Although more than pleased to be shot of the Royal Navy in 1948, there were some aspects of it which I missed. I often yearned to be at sea again, just watching the sea in all its moods, feeling the keen wind and experiencing a primal contact with the eternal things – the clouds, the pure air, the horizons, the albatrosses, the dolphins, whales and the flying fishes. So instead of an air journey we splashed out on a first-class stateroom on the Union Castle Line flagship, the RMS *Windsor Castle*, for the two-and-a-half day sea trip from Southampton to Las Palmas in the Canary Islands. I was agog at the prospect of a sea journey once more, some thirty years after my final sea voyage in the Navy, the troopship from Freetown in 1945. B was just as excited, never having voyaged by sea. We had the whole nostalgic bit – the boat train from Waterloo Station, the excitement of boarding at Southampton, an iced lager in the first-class saloon, the actual departure with booming sirens and miles of ribbons between ship and shore, the innumerable photographs and the excitement and the waving and the tears. We were soon down the Solent and past the Isle of Wight when I was slowly overwhelmed by a crushing disappointment. I discovered that a large modern liner is not a bit like a naval vessel – high out of the water, so *aloof* from the sea itself – it felt just like a large floating hotel; which it was, of course. Silly me to have expected otherwise. The great thing hardly rolled at all, and there was very little pitching. No rising and falling of the bows, no feeling of the sea being only a few feet away, as on even the largest of battleships. It was one of the biggest let-downs of my life – and all that money for the luxury of it. I felt on the point of issuing a writ against the Union Castle Line for misrepresentation. So we just settled down and enjoyed the life of Riley for a couple of days, including the Captain's cocktail party and stumbling across two delightful geriatric Americans – Ethel and Sam – who became bosom friends and were the most tremendous fun. It was quite a wrench to say goodbye and go down the gangway to Las Palmas. We met them many times after that, in London, since they were inveterate travellers. They are both gone now. May their merry souls rest in peace – we love them still.

I should describe here how the interest, sponsorship and patronage of one senior Consultant Orthopaedic Surgeon, namely Mr Peter Newington CBE DSO MC FRCS, of the Royal National Orthopaedic Hospital in London, helped smooth the path of developing joint manipulation treatments, by physiotherapists, in NHS hospitals. He was influential in advocating my appointment as a Clinical Tutor at RNOH and I am sure that his advocacy influenced his consultant colleagues.

Mr Newington enthusiastically lectured on the annual long courses, sponsored by the Chartered Society of Physiotherapy and held at RNOH. The development of the courses was a direct result of his patronage being made manifest to the orthopaedic and rheumatology worlds.

The fifties and sixties were a time of change anyway and many factors, which we need not consider here, were operating to change doctors' prescriptions of physiotherapy from 'Heat and exercises three times a week for one month' to the simple 'Physiotherapy, please', thus leaving decisions about the nature and duration of treatment to the physiotherapist.

Other than manipulation under anaesthesia by orthopaedic surgeons, which was common in all large hospitals, in the majority of them the physiotherapy departments did not offer joint manipulation of the conscious patient as an accepted part of the treatment. There was probably only one hospital – St Thomas's of London – which gave its physiotherapy students regular instruction in manipulation of spinal and peripheral joints. This instruction at STH was initiated in earlier days by Dr J.B. Marlowe, and continued during the forties by Dr J. Carfax, who introduced a well-constructed and logical system of examination, together with a somewhat different system of techniques. Many physiotherapy teachers of other hospitals, who had completed manipulation courses by Dr Carfax at St Thomas's hospital, became enthusiastic about the clarity and logic of his teaching, and taught the principles to their own students. Also, for some considerable time, Dr Carfax's senior physiotherapists had conducted teaching courses at home and abroad. Yet it was true to say that it was not usual for consultants in Rheumatology and Orthopaedics to expect that their physiotherapy staffs were competent and capable in the matter of joint manipulation. Further, not all consultants dealing with neuro-musculo-skeletal conditions were enthusiastic about Dr Carfax's approach.

However, the clinical climate was changing, and physiotherapists trained in manipulative techniques began to influence their peers and colleagues, changing the nature and scale of treatment available for common joint conditions in the physiotherapy departments of NHS hospitals and in private practice. Mr Peter Newington's advocacy exerted a considerable influence in bringing about this clinical climatic change.

By now Barbara was as deeply involved as I was – in our own time. She typed the minutes of meetings, and lecture notes, and course programmes, plus letters to the multitude of correspondents at home and abroad, especially Canada, the USA and Australia. I was still teaching at every opportunity; we went to Liverpool four times, for example. I vividly recall picking B up from her work on a Friday evening at 5.30 and then haring up the Edgware Road to the M1, and then the M6, munching Marks and Spencer pork pies and tomatoes in the car as we pressed northwards. One night at about 11.00 p.m., we had a rear tyre blow-out on the M6; I was doing about 80 m.p.h. and had it been a front tyre we would have been for it. I managed to control the car, a little Renault Ten, and having changed the wheel we pressed on and completed the weekend of teaching. We drove home on the Sunday evening and started the week's work on the Monday morning. This went on for four years.

I had also instituted the 'RNOH Evenings', a monthly series of informal lectures spread over three years. There was no administration and there were no fees. They were exciting times. I would stand up in the lecture theatre and start talking at 6.00 p.m. on the first Thursday of each month, going on until about 7.15 or later if the interest was still there, which it sometimes was. They were not always lectures, although I had chosen a subject which fitted into a progressive scheme. They sometimes developed into discussions. Anybody who felt like it could raise points for discussion or even go off at a tangent if the assembly seemed agreeable. An astonishing number of knotty points were raised, and the unusual format seemed to generate its own popularity. I proudly recall one of the junior Registrars asking how many the lecture theatre could seat. Came the reply: 'Ask Mr Grieve – he fills it on the first Thursday of every month.' It was immensely gratifying to note that some had travelled considerable distances to attend the talks. I know the jokes were pretty good but they weren't that good, so it must have been the clinical content. This went on for three years, while we steadfastly churned out a 20-25 page 'Newsletter' every two months, which carried original articles from home and overseas, especially the translations of some excellent German Manual Therapy writers. We were fortunate to enjoy the willing and cost-free services of my old physiotherapy school classmate, Peter Cooper. He had an external degree in Modern Languages, i.e. French, German and Russian, and for many years kept us well up-to-date with what was happening on the Continent, so far as our speciality was concerned. We continued to conduct the affairs of the Manipulation Association of Chartered Physiotherapists, a rapidly expanding body of therapists who had satisfied demanding entry requirements. The 1973, 1974 and 1975 courses at Great Portland Street got progressively more complex and ambitious, with two other teachers, Cynthia Merrill and Philip Woods, joining to help carry the load. Facilities at the Royal National Orthopaedic Hospital were excellent. The lecture theatre was commodious and very well equipped. I was free to enjoy the excellent services of the Photographic Department and was relieved of actual clinical duties during the course teaching times. It became possible to include teaching by some of the best orthopaedic men in the country. RNOH Consultants in Orthopaedics Neurology, Rheumatology and other specialities happily agreed to give course lectures – the standard of instruction was very high indeed. Both the Superintendent and Assistant Super-intendent of the Norfolk and Norwich hospital came down to London for the courses and I was pleased to see a strong East Anglian presence among the candidates. The link with East Anglia was strengthened when two of the Registrars at RNOH became Orthopaedic Consultants at the N and N Hospital in Norwich.

Being of an enquiring mind and therefore glad to make use of whatever sources of information were available to me, I had a field day in the Institute of Orthopaedics Library, part of the Royal National Orthopaedic Hospital. The library was a veritable treasure house. The range of texts, and particularly of journals and periodicals, was breathtaking, including many of the classical journals going back to the year dot. I happily plunged in, and soon evolved my own system of background reading – which went on all the time – and of scanning the journals as they came in. I would sift through each new arrival, photocopying the title page of anything which interested me, then pass the pages to a secretary, who would compose a standard letter of request for reprints to each author. The early stream of papers and reprints steadily became a torrent, needing much time for reading, sorting and filing. I devised a somewhat idiosyncratic alphabetical filing system, initially of some forty-eight foolscap boxes, together with a system of sequential numbering as the boxes filled up. 'Anatomy', for example, grew as 'A1', 'A11', and 'A111' and so on. 'Upper Cervical Spine' grew as 'U1', 'U11' and 'U111'. The individual papers were also numbered sequentially, of course, as 'A1', 'A2' and 'A3'. By referring to the Master List I could put my hand on any paper at a moment's notice. Without any training in librarianship, which is a highly technical subject, I seemed to have an indexing type of mind, and by following the dictates of my instincts just fell into a logical way of progressing. The foolscap boxes were labelled, for example, as Anatomy, Adjunct Treatments, Anomalies, Autonomic Nervous System, Backache-Treatment and Management, Biomechanics, Bone-Physiology and Pathology, Cervical Spine Pathology (the highly important cranio-vertebral junction papers were filed under 'U' – Upper Cervical Spine), Diagnostic Procedures and Investigations, Disc Pathology, Examination and Assessment, Function of Joints and Muscles, Lifting and Handling, Manipulation, Manipulation Accidents, Neurology, Pain and Referred Pain, Pathology of Thoracic Spine and Ribs, Pathology of Lumbar Spine, Prophylaxis, Psychology of Spinal Pain, Sacro-iliac Joint, Space-occupying Lesions, Treatment Philosophies, and so on. It was a highly individual system, and I knew just where everything was. The system had the advantage of being flexible enough to absorb any amount of new material efficiently and without being overwhelmed. It just needed more and more space although it is surprising how much can be squirrelled away and yet remain instantly accessible, so long as all containers are of a standard size and shape. I flattered myself that so long as a newcomer had access to the Master List, any paper could be quickly located after a scan of the List.

I also subscribed to some twenty other sources, either on my own account or as Editor of our Association's 'Newsletter'. Among these were the following publications:

Physiotherapy, Manuelle Medizin (German), *Journal of Bone and Joint Surgery* British and American issues, *Journal of Orthopaedic and Sports Physical Therapy, Australian Manipulative Therapists' News,* British Association of Manipulative Medicine *Newsletter,* Canadian Manual Therapy Group *Newsletter,* Medical Research Council *News,* Journal of Eular – *European League Against Rheumatism,* Proceedings of Australian Manual Therapy Group Congresses, the journal *Spine, Physiotherapy Practice, British Osteopathic Journal* and bibliographies of the American, Canadian, New Zealand, Australian and South African physiotherapy journals. Just as the air is stuffed with all kinds of electro-magnetic radiations, so the clinical world is awash with information. Keeping abreast of it requires application and organization.

I digressed here to talk about the marshalling of information, since I had begun to devote my energies to producing texts for newcomers to the interest. I could not contemplate this without an information base, a database. The 1975 paperback facsimile of Barbara's type-written pages – *Mobilisation of the Spine* – which I mentioned earlier, went into successive editions in 1977 and 1979. The third edition was given professional clothes by the medical publisher, Messrs Churchill Livingstone of Edinburgh. It later went on to 4th and 5th editions, the latter going into several reprints. This was encouraging, and as I had begun to get my writing published in the journal *Physiotherapy* from

1958 onwards, I felt the urge to set my sights on a more ambitious textbook.

It is said that inspiration is the art of applying the seat of the pants, with determination, to the seat of the chair. But the Regent's Park area of London is so beguiling. Since the Medical Research Council inhabits Park Crescent W1, Barbara was fortunate enough to work behind a gracefully curved Nash facade. She much enjoyed her time there and made a host of friends. We used to walk down Albany Street to work, she to the MRC and me to RNOH. We loved equally the grace of the beautiful Nash terraces and the raffishly decadent air of Camden High Street and its environs, which I'd first encountered on attending the Crowndale Working Men's College in 1949. The region is full of history and interest; the liver-coloured tiles of Mornington Crescent Underground station, the graceful Harley Street, Cavendish Street, Weymouth Street and Marylebone High Street. Not far away was Fitzroy Street – 'Fitzrovia' – with the studios of the painters Frith ('Derby Day') Whistler and Sickert. Much of Sickert's best work was produced there, as were the 'Fitzroy Street Nudes' of the Fauvist Matthew Smith. I had read much of Sickert, not only of his life and his paintings but of his writings, too, since he wielded a lively pen and was forever firing off letters to *The Times* and other papers. In 1947, MacMillan published *A Free House or The Artist As Craftsman*, a collection of his writings.

Barbara and I used to just wander about the fairly large area covered by the Euston Road, Fitzroy Street and Camden High Street identifying buildings such as the house where Dickens's illustrator Cruikshank, used to live. Also Granby Street, where Sickert painted so many of those lovely *contre jour* nudes, and the site of the Old Bedford Music Hall in Camden. Sickert often painted there during performances, especially of the faces peering over the edges of the boxes. There was a delightful air of dusty, faded Edwardian elegance about Mornington Crescent, Camden Town and the more up-market Park Villages – East and West. The whole area was redolent with the now fading signatures of a more elegant 'times past' which seemed only just to have gone. When one got tired of the Nash terraces of polyglot Camden Town there was always Regent's Park, one of the more delightful of London's open spaces. It was even possible to get a good view of the elephant house of the zoo from a slight rise of the ground – without paying to go in.

Not far away was the Pentonville Road, from the high rise of which John O'Connor had painted that beautiful misty evening vista of *St. Pancras Hotel and Station from Pentonville Road: Sunset* (1884). The whole region was immortalized in the paintings of Robert Bevan, Charles Ginner, Harold Gilman, Spencer Gore and of Sickert, of course. There is a beautifully understated view of London chimney pots, from a Harley Street window, painted in 1948 by Mary Potter. So much of Camden Town, Hampstead, Islington and 'Fitzrovia' still speaks of those painters of the short-lived Camden Town Group during the years 1905-14, although Mary Potter was not one of these.

Dating from an introductory course I'd conducted in 1969 at the Norfolk and Norwich hospital, a seed had certainly been sown, and my links with East Anglia were strengthened by the two and a bit years I had spent at Oldchurch Hospital in Romford. It became evident that a welcome awaited me in Norwich, should B and I decide to uproot and move to East

Anglia. We were both beginning to weary of the unremitting, incessant pressure, of running the courses, producing the Newsletter, teaching here, there and everywhere, gathering material for a book and formulating its skeletal framework, preparing the 'RNOH Evening' lectures and other commitments, plus the never-ending stream of patients at RNOH. There were several pointers to a watershed – we were approaching the tenth anniversary of the founding of the Manipulation Association. I had been awarded an Honorary Fellowship of the Chartered Society in 1975 and the younger ones were now coming along. Barbara had reached retiring age. The International Federation of Orthopaedic Manipulative Physiotherapists had been formed in Montreal in 1974, and I had begun to feel it was time to start allocating more of my energies, and those of Barbara, to producing a book, something more ambitious than a little paperback. At the end of each weekend at the cottages in Cratfield, it was becoming harder and harder to pile into the car and drive back to London. During 1975 we decided it was time to make a move in the next year. We sold the cottages in 1975 and moved our East Anglian possessions into our home-to-be in Halesworth. In March 1976 we shook the dust of London from our feet – not without some pain – to settle in East Anglia. It really did seem like coming home.

This was on the promise of a Vice-Principal's salary for two days a week at the N and N Hospital, while we began a Private Clinic for three days a week in Halesworth, some twenty-five miles from Norwich. I had some very good friends in the town – two of the Orthopaedic Consultants, the Superintendent Physiotherapist and her Assistant, and the Superintendent of one of the Ipswich hospitals. We also had firm friends in Cratfield, and for many years had felt like natives rather than foreigners.

As the furniture van pulled away from Park Village East with our few bits and pieces of a small London flat, we packed Barbara's favourite little electric stove into our small Renault Five and got a scratch meal before turning in, preparatory to clearing the flat in the morning and driving to Suffolk. Neither of us could sleep a wink! At about 2.30 in the morning we said 'What the hell!' got some breakfast and drove through a quiet, sleeping London to Suffolk. We stopped in a lay-by just before Halesworth and had a short sleep in the car. After a cup of coffee from the vacuum flask we drove on to our new home. The place we stopped was henceforth known as 'Sleep lay-by".

Having, some months earlier, discussed with the Chartered Society of Physiotherapy that I would be relinquishing responsibility for the long courses after 1975, there was a certain careless rapture during our first two weeks at 'Hill Drive' in Halesworth, before I took up my part-time post at the Norwich Hospital. I was free of London now, although B and I kept responsibility for the newsletter. Local builders were still rehabilitating some of the rooms of our Edwardian bungalow, and laying some 100 yards of the drive, but the kitchen, bathroom and the future treatment room were quite habitable. We moved in, in a kind of limbo – having left London but not yet fully arrived in Suffolk. It felt much the same as when I was in the US Army camp in Casablanca in 1943, having survived the sinking of a troopship – a limbo of no responsibility and of no demands to be met, in this case for at least two or three weeks.

Three weeks later, I began part-time work as a Clinical Tutor in the Physical Medicine (Rheumatology) Department of the Norfolk and Norwich Hospital. It was the beginning of a very happy three years. I was among friends and got on well with the Consultant Rheumatologist, Dr G. Winstanley. Both the Superintendent Physiotherapist and her Deputy had come down to London as candidates on the Long Manipulation Courses during the early seventies, and two of the N and N Consultant Orthopaedic Surgeons – Harold Phelps and Kenneth Tuckson – had been friendly Orthopaedic Registrar colleagues during my years at the Royal National Orthopaedic Hospital in London.

I worked at the N and N Hospital for two days a week and started a private manipulative practice in Halesworth on Mondays, Wednesdays and Fridays. It was a strange beginning – Barbara and I would be working in the garden when the phone went. Barbara offered an appointment within the hour while I hastily tidied up, changed into a clinical-looking white jacket and stood in the treatment room ready to receive the patient, looking as though I'd been doing nothing else all morning.

The hospital lay some twenty-five miles north of Halesworth, and was reached by a pleasant drive through wheatfields, through the little market town of Bungay and then across the river Waveney which divided Norfolk and Suffolk. During that prolonged dry summer of 1976 East Anglia shared in the general drought conditions. I recall driving home one evening while the dusty cornfields were being harvested, with the air thick with corndust as the combine harvesters pushed their way through the wheat. It was quite difficult to breathe comfortably, and a great relief to reach Halesworth and get clear of the dusty fields.

My days were more interesting than Barbara's. She had abruptly changed from a high-powered, demanding occupation at the Medical Research Council to being virtually housebound as a clinical practice housewife, whose main duties, apart from running the house, were to make appointments for the patients. I know there were times when her hours seemed to hang heavily, and for that reason I phoned her several times during my hospital days, and that helped, she said. As so often in the past, she had happily modified her life and interests to serve mine. I was a fortunate man. Yet she was truly interested in the work, and derived a great deal of satisfaction from seeing the results of our working together. As the practice grew, which it quickly did, she became much busier and more involved, both as 'practice manager' and 'accountant' and also as clinical assistant in the treatment room. She became adept at keeping the appointment book full, with the work evenly spaced out. I was always pleased that in all of our endeavours it was just Barbara and I working together. Whether we were rehabilitating our cottages, doing some gardening, producing the books, conducting the practice and so on, we always worked beautifully together. When both going for the same thing, we used to go like a bomb. A second assistant would have been unthinkable, and it used to give me great pleasure to acknowledge, in my books, that she was the other half of the team.

It was fortunate for me that my old boss at RNOH in London, the Consultant Orthopaedic Surgeon Peter Newington, had retired to Aldeburgh – some eight miles away on the coast – and was an important and influential member of the local golf club. A number of my earliest patients had attended my clinic on his recommendation and this gave the practice a good start locally. I had also taken the trouble to write to, and visit, all General Practitioners within twenty-five miles of my house, thereby making myself known over a sizeable portion of my own neck of the woods. I had a cordial relationship too with the Aldeburgh GPs, who knew that their patients would be carefully and responsibly handled. My contacting the GPs had taken an immense amount of old-fashioned legwork, but it paid off handsomely in the end.

Meanwhile Barbara had slowly checked every single square yard of the big garden (almost an acre of it) which had been virtually unattended during the period when the house was for sale. She had found some wild snake's head fritillaries, which we carefully fostered. It was lovely to see them appear every spring thereafter. We laid the garden as hedges and lawns, since there was no way we would have had the time for horticulture of almost an acre of garden. By dint of getting enough equipment, and making an electrical power outlet at one end of the grounds, I was able to grass-cut and hedge-trim, gaining a certain satisfaction in managing to cope on my own. Since we had a mower for Barbara, too, she often pitched in and joined the party.

I had begun to get my writing published in *Physio-therapy* from 1958 onwards, and the success enjoyed by my little paperback was prompting me to do more ambitious things. By moving lock, stock and barrel to Suffolk I seemed to pave the way to seriously start writing again, to raise my sights and begin thinking about a full-blown textbook on the speciality. Manipulative physiotherapists in other countries had begun to produce texts of different kinds and the prospect was plainly in the air in many countries.

I had already had some experience writing comprehensively, in this case on the sacro-iliac joint. During late 1975 and 1976, I had been working on an article about this interesting joint – largely because I felt my knowledge of it was patchy and one of the best ways of learning about something is to have to explain it, or teach it, to others. During 1976 I continued developing the material to the point where it comprised enough to provide copy for two *Physiotherapy* journal articles. I submitted the MS to the Journal Editor late in that year when it was proposed that both sections should be published in the one issue for December 1976. This was even more encouraging, and I began to conceive a comprehensive framework for a full-blown text on spinal joint problems ('Common Vertebral Joint Problems'). I planned to incorporate General and Regional Anatomy, Structural Anomalies, Pathological Changes (General and Regional), Forms of Clinical Presentation, Incidence (Regional and General), Clinical Features, Examination, Assessment and Investigation Procedures (X-rays, myelograms, etc.), Treatment Techniques, Indications and Contraindications, Adjunct Treatments, Conditions requiring a Surgical Opinion and so on. There were many more subject headings, of course, but the foregoing gives an idea of how I had planned the project. It was ambitious but I was sure I could do it. I finished the MS in 1979 and delivered it to the publisher's office in London. Churchill Livingstone had agreed to take it on and the first edition was published in 1981. The book was reprinted in 1983, 1984 and 1985 and was short-listed for the 1983 Abbott Prize for Medical Writing. B and I were quite delighted with this response and began enjoying the financial results of those years of toil and hope.

After coping with the winter driving of 1978/79, I became weary of the often hazardous 25-mile journey to Norwich and back. The roads were not as wide in places as they might be and the going was often treacherous and dangerous. Accordingly, I relinquished my post at the N and N Hospital in March 1979 and concentrated my efforts at the Halesworth practice. There was a certain enjoyable freedom in having the flexibility of time to arrange patient appointments according only to clinical need – some weeks we worked for six days and on other weeks only for two or three. And I didn't have to drive a motor car to work. I still visited the hospital to give the occasional lecture, and once a month sat in on Mr Phelps's Wednesday morning Orthopaedic Clinic; they were pure pleasure. We would look at patients together, formulating our diagnostic opinions and deciding on treatment. The follow-up appointments were arranged to coincide with my next visit. I always found Mr Phelps's company agreeable and they were very happy occasions.

In July of 1982 Churchill Livingstone invited me to compile and edit an international text on Manual Therapy. I was not sure the publisher realized just how much of a blockbuster it would have to be. As eventually mentioned in the Preface, the publisher's invitation prompted my first concept of a rich and comprehensive totality. Constraints of the possible soon whittled down that vision, yet the remaining 85 chapters, written by 61 authors from 9 countries were, I hoped, a fair representation of what physiotherapists were thinking and doing in the mid-eighties, together with authoritative accounts of some contexts of that work. The countries represented were Australia, Canada, Czechoslovakia, Denmark, New Zealand, South Africa, Sweden, United Kingdom and the USA. The book was published in the autumn of 1986, and enjoyed five printings.

I was also invited to prepare a second edition of *Common Vertebral Joint Problems*, which we got stuck into almost at once. This was published to coincide with the 1988 Congress at Cambridge of the International Federation of Orthopaedic Manipulative Therapists. Soon after that B and I completed the 5th edition of my little paperback, now a hefty handful – that, too, went into three printings.

We were both beginning to long for a more sedate existence. The demands of patients, the paperwork and the letters to the doctors had all begun to take their toll. Writing is the hardest work in the world not involving heavy lifting. Barbara had typed herself to a standstill and I had taught, and written, myself to a standstill. In 1990 we decided we had had enough. We were going to opt for some peace and quiet. We closed the practice.

It was a lovely summer that year – day after day of blue sky and sun. We had a ball giving the house a fresh-up. Barbara steadily washed every curtain and blanket in sight and I steadily decorated the kitchen, main bedroom, sitting room and hall. We really spread sideways, as it were, in the happy release from drudgery and deadlines. I donated over 1,200 teaching slides to a London hospital physiotherapy school, and gave all my books and some thousands of indexed papers to the library of the Manipulation Association of Chartered Physiotherapists. At different times, one or other of the books were translated into one of six languages: French, Dutch, Portuguese, Spanish, Greek and Japanese – and the royalties kept coming in March of each year.

We had some fifteen months of retired happiness together, before the next inevitable milestone hove into view. We could look back on a prodigious amount of work, mostly unpaid and in our own time – for our own reasons – and derived immense satisfaction from what we had achieved. Barbara was quite superb in her administrative capacities. Pre-war she had been a civil servant at the Post Office Savings headquarters in London, where she absorbed an excellent training in clerical and administrative organization. When the publisher proposed a second edition of what was now to be called *Grieve's Modern Manual Therapy of the Vertebral Column*, this was after B had died, and the two new editors suggested that the book be dedicated to Barbara's memory. I quote:

> The Editors have kindly suggested that this edition be dedicated to Barbara Grieve, whose secretarial expertise and administrative skills contributed so much to the successful production of the first edition. In total and loving commitment she energetically devoted herself to achieving the very best presentation of the final manuscript – everything passing through her hands being thoroughly organised and impeccably turned out on her faithful portable typewriter. Having taken a lively interest in my training as a physiotherapist she had the wit to perceive the great potential of neuro-musculo-skeletal medicine. Her enthusiastic efforts to further the welfare of the Manipulation Association of Chartered Physiotherapists also embraced the aims of the International Federation of Orthopaedic Manipulative Therapists. Like the CSP Manipulation courses in the early days to 1975, the MACP

and the IFOMT have handsomely acknowledged how much they owe to her.

While she deprecated her talents as those of a self-taught amateur, her considerable achievements truly were a labour of love, as well as of genuine interest in the work. She was the other half of the team, and she warmed whoever was associated with her. She has left a little of herself in so many hearts, world-wide.

In August of 1991, she had begun to find difficulty in fine movements of her right hand. It gradually became obvious that her musculo-skeletal function was progressively being affected. She began to develop muscular weakness, and during September and October had several falls. I would go into a room and find her crumpled on the floor, unable to get herself up. One day she seemed to take a long time to walk up the drive, and I went out to find her fallen into a hawthorn hedge. She was admitted to the West Norwich Hospital for neurological assessment, and was diagnosed as suffering from a progressive illness of the nervous system – this was already manifest, of course. She spent the last week of her life in the Halesworth Patrick Stead Hospital. Three days before she died she made the great effort to lift her hand and stroke my face – she was saying goodbye. I had been with her throughout the night of 19/20 November, and watched her peacefully die in the early morning of the 20th. I had lost my life's companion and my true love. All I can do is soldier on and finish my own course with as much dignity as I can muster. I looked back over our achievements. We had given much, I think, and had enjoyed the privilege of doing so.

Bibliography

1. Morgan, B. (Ed.), *The Great Trains* (Lausanne, Edita, 1973).
2. Biddle, G., Nock, O.S., *The Railway Heritage of Britain* (London, Michael Joseph, 1983).
3. Mondey, D. (Ed.), *International Encyclopaedia of Aviation* (London, Octopus Books, 1977).
4. Thompson, K., *HMS* Rodney *at War* (London, Hollis and Carter, 1946).
5. McMurtrie, F., *The Cruise of the* Bismarck (London, Hutchinson and Co., 1946).
6. Gray, E., *Hitler's Battleships* (London, Leo Cooper, 1972).
7. Coles, A., Briggs, E., *Flagship Hood* (London, Hale, 1985).
8. Van der Vet, D., *The Atlantic Campaign* (London, Hodder & Stoughton, 1988).
9. Raven, A., Roberts, J., *British Battleships of World War Two* (London, Arms & Armour Press, 1976).
10. Raven, A., Roberts, J., *British Cruisers of World War Two* (London, Arms & Armour Press, 1980).
11. Smith, P.C., *The Great Ships Pass* (London, W. Kimber, 1977).

12. Costello, J., Hughes, T., *The Battle of the Atlantic* (London, Collins, 1977).
13. Keegan, J., *The Second World War* (London, Hutchinson, 1989).
14. Von Mullenheim-Rechberg, B., *Battleship* Bismarck – *A Survivor's Story* (London, Bodley Head, 1980).
15. Kennedy, L., *Pursuit – The Chase and Sinking of the* Bismarck (London, Collins, 1974).
16. Hough, R., *Dreadnought – A History of the Modern Battleship* (London, Michael Joseph, 1965).
17. Ireland, B., Gibbons, T., *Jane's Battleships of the 20th Century* (London, Harper Collins, 1996).
18. Hill, J.R. (Ed.), *Oxford Illustrated History of the Royal Navy* (Oxford, University Press, 1995).
19. Lamb, C., *To War in a Stringbag* (London, Nelson Doubleday, 1980).
20. Fairbanks, D. (Jr.), *A Hell of a War* (London, Robson Books, 1995).
21. Woodward, D., *Tirpitz* (London, New English Library, 1974).
22. Shepherd, C., *German Aircraft of World War II* (London, Book Club Associates, 1975).
23. Frayn Turner, J., *British Aircraft of World War II* (London, Book Club Associates, 1975).
24. Elfrath, U., Herzog, B., *The Battleship* Bismarck (Westchester, Pennsylvania, Schiffer Publishing, 1989).
25. McMurtrie, F.E., *Jane's Fighting Ships 1931* (Newton Abbot, Devon, David & Charles Reprints, 1973).
26. Gross, J., *The Oxford Book of Aphorisms* (Oxford, University Press, 1983).
27. Harris, A., *Bomber Offensive* (London, Collins, 1947).

28. Barnett, C., *Engage the Enemy More Closely – The Royal Navy in the Second World War* (London, Hodder & Stoughton, 1991).